The Bastard Tree

A Memoir

Carol Holoboff

iUniverse, Inc.
New York Bloomington

The Bastard Tree

A Memoir

Copyright © 2008 by Carol Holoboff

All rights reserved. No part of this book may be used or reproduced by any means, graphic, electronic, or mechanical, including photocopying, recording, taping or by any information storage retrieval system without the written permission of the publisher except in the case of brief quotations embodied in critical articles and reviews.

The views expressed in this work are solely those of the author and do not necessarily reflect the views of the publisher, and the publisher hereby disclaims any responsibility for them.

iUniverse books may be ordered through booksellers or by contacting:

iUniverse
1663 Liberty Drive
Bloomington, IN 47403
www.iuniverse.com
1-800-Authors (1-800-288-4677)

Because of the dynamic nature of the Internet, any Web addresses or links contained in this book may have changed since publication and may no longer be valid. The views expressed in this work are solely those of the author and do not necessarily reflect the views of the publisher, and the publisher hereby disclaims any responsibility for them.

ISBN: 978-0-595-53474-6 (pbk)
ISBN: 978-0-595-63532-0 (ebk)

Printed in the United States of America

iUniverse rev. date: 11/25/2008

Also by Carol Holoboff

Camp Francis for Every Community

For Dr. William Taylor, who thought me virtuous

Table of Contents

Roots 1
The Rodeo 15
Peacetime 23
The Making Of An Orphan 35
St. Thomas 43
Me And Grandma 53
Continental Divides 65
Helena Valley 73
Sweet Grass 83
Gardner 93
The Banich Family 101
Astoria 115
The Cuckoo Lands 123
The Holly Family 135
The Lapin Family 143
The Holoboffs 147
Coming Out Of Chute #2 159
Camp Francis 169
Conclusion 177
Epilogue 179

"It is never to late to be what you might have been."

George Eliot

Acknowledgments

I have had the good fortune to find a mentor and a friend in Gordon Sullivan, who prodded and pulled me along on those days when I was discouraged and celebrated the successful steps I made in the long process of putting my story to paper. I also want thank Ruth McLaughlin for seven years of encouragement, availability, and unconditional regard. Special thanks to Marylou Holoboff for reading the manuscript and asking questions that went unanswered in the first draft. The ladies of the Libby writer's group deserve more than a thank you for sitting through repeated readings of the same story rewritten many times. They were always positive, supportive, and they laughed only in the right places. I mention Chris Caubel, the only publisher who got the chance to reject my manuscript, because he took the time to read the first very rough draft and then wrote an encouraging letter that showed he had indeed read it all. Without friends like Sandy McGuffin and Kathy Lacunza who may not have thought I could do it, but never said so, I might have given up. Thank you will never be enough for my children who lived the story and are willing to let me tell it and finally, my everlasting gratitude to Sydney, my husband, my friend and my partner, who has allowed me to write the ugly parts of our story and has stayed around for the "the best is yet to be" part.

Introduction

Sometimes a life happens, even when no one is paying attention. This is a story about a life that happened. There are those who need to know what happened during my seventy years of life and there are those who think they know but really don't. Names have not been changed to protect the innocent; none were, but they must be forgiven.

You may have passed by our house last Thanksgiving and looked through the lace curtains at the family gathered around the holiday table. You may have thought we were just "regular" folks. I hope you did. It was the first Thanksgiving in thirty years that we were together. We came through unspeakable experiences and un-measurable sadness to form the unique circle that defines our family.

Holidays are marking days for families. Stories, told and retold, become family legends. Those who have heard them before savor them, and new members listen in wonder. Other stories drift through the day unspoken, but are shared nonetheless. Some of those unspoken stories are silenced by shame or regret but all family circles vibrate with some kind of change: deaths and divorces, weddings and births, friendship and betrayal, but those circles still exist.

On the eastern side of the continental divide wind spills over granite peaks and thunders onto the foothills. They pick up speed and scream across Montana's prairie, taking with them anything not deeply rooted. Although my roots were shallow I somehow hung on and by pressing my face against other windows framed with lace curtains of normalcy,

I learned the imposter's lines and found my way from white trash to white collar. My story must be given voice so our unique family circle won't be broken again.

CHAPTER 1—ROOTS

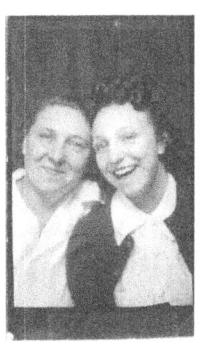

I once asked my sister Margaret, who was fourteen years old when I was born in 1938, if I had been an accident. She angrily insisted that Mother had adored me. However, mostly, the mother of my memories, consumed in her quest to keep a roof over our heads, was impatient and quick to anger.

That's my half-sister, Margaret in the picture with Mother. She was pretty. She had dark curly hair and skin that looked like porcelain. They had the picture taken in one of those photo booths at the state fair. That is how I remember them, comfortable together.

Just weeks before she died, Mother and I rode the Ferris wheel at the state fair. When we stopped at the wheel's highest point we clung to the wooden crossbar as our chair rocked. I leaned forward to look down at the busy midway and Mother grabbed the back of my shirt and pulled me close. We looked out past the grandstand and horse barns, beyond the fairgrounds and across the river. It seemed we were no longer part of the world below. I watched the Merry-Go-Round steeds rise and fall in time with the calliope music and I caught whiffs cotton candy from below. We swooped round and round on the giant erector-set wheel and time seemed to stand still. Then it was our turn to get off.

On the back of my sister's picture are the words, "Mom and I at the fair," as though even a half century later, there could be no mistake who the "I" was. After Margaret and I were grown, she still referred to our mother in conversation as "my" mother, and I left her claim unchallenged.

I was born on July 19, and my parents brought me home from Deaconess Hospital on the city bus. Paperboys stood on street corners with stacks of orange-colored afternoon newspapers and called out the headlines. A decade later I would sing from my own corner, "Get your Great Falls paper, Leader, read all about it," but that hot summer afternoon, I was the big news at the Davenport Hotel.

My first home was a one-room flat in a brick tenement above the Lobby Bar. Neighbors sat at their windows with their curtains tied back to catch a breeze in the hot afternoon and watched the activity two stories below on Central Avenue. They waved and shouted when they saw my parents get off the bus with me. Mother probably blushed at the attention. She was quite a bit older than her young neighbors who were youthfully attractive even in their shapeless housedresses and rolled-down stockings.

My dad's mother, Grandma Johnson, said mother was what people might call a handsome woman. "Sturdy, you know," she would add in a catty mother-in-law way.

Grandma said Mother kept her eyes on the worn linoleum as they family passed through a gauntlet of "oohs" and "aahs" on the way to our room, but Daddy stopped at each doorway so the ladies could get a better look at me. I was my Daddy's first and only child and, although he was wearing his ever-present fedora, which made him almost as tall as Mother, he was walking taller that day because of my birth. Daddy was just barely five foot eight but he claimed he always wore the hat because someone might want to purchase one of his special hand-tied fishing flies that were hooked in the hatband.

Both of my parents were both born in October in the year nineteen-ought-one, as folks used to say, but they were born continents apart. Mother was born in Austria and she came through Ellis Island with her mother in 1906. My dad and his dad too, were born in the tiny coal-mining town of Belt, Montana.

Mother's father came to the new country without his pregnant girl friend and it took him over five years to pay for their passage. The Urban family stayed in Cleveland, Ohio for a short time before migrating to

Montana. They lived in Cline, a settlement of houses on the outskirts of Roundup that belonged to the coal mine.

Mother—Victoria and Rudolph's only child—learned to speak English when she started school in Roundup. She asked her parents not to call her Milka, their pet name for her, in front of her friends. So, Amelia became Millie, and her parents watched with immigrant pride as their daughter graduated from Roundup High School. But then their "thoroughly modern Millie" rushed wildly into the roaring twenties. I saw a picture of her when she was about 17 dressed like a flapper, cloche hat, short no-waist dress and white stockings. She was laughing in the photograph as she leaned toward the camera in a flirty pose.

Mother married before she was twenty. Walter, Paul and Margaret Pollock were my half brothers and sister. When Mother was twenty-four she was divorced and Mr. Pollock took Walter and Paul back to Ohio. Mother kept Margaret with her and worked as a cook on ranches in the Great Falls area. She married again in 1929 but that marriage ended in 1934 and there were no children from that marriage. My mother and father were married in 1937.

Grandpa Urban worked until he was sixty-eight and then had to apply for assistance from the United Mine Workers of America's Welfare and Retirement Fund. His disability was listed as "chronic bronchitis." Victoria Urban died when she was ninety-three. Her legacy to me was a mayonnaise jar full of coins. It was December of 1972. I was a single mother of four and I worked nights in a convenience store. I managed to pay our bills but there was little money left over for extras and it was almost Christmas. Every time I checked the mailbox the kids would tease me about my "ship" that hadn't come in yet. I didn't even know my grandmother was still alive. My brother Walter found our address in Oregon and one day there was my ship in the mailbox. The package contained a glass jar that was packed tight in popcorn. Inside the jar were $43.24 and a note written in another language. My brother had translated the note; "Give this money to little Carol." My grandmother had saved her widow's mite for me in a jar that the family found when they cleaned out her belongings. The kids had a nice Christmas and learned a little about faith.

My dad's mother traveled from Missouri with her mother, a new stepfather and several full and half-siblings sometime before the turn of the twentieth century. They came to claim their 640 acres under the 1877 Desert Land Act. They hoped to fulfill the requirement that they irrigate the land within three years in order to claim it. The Bell boys got their start in Montana because some of my grandma's brothers were able to keep their land.

For many years I assumed my grandma's name was Clarabelle, but actually it was Carrie Bell. She married Walter Johnson in 1900 when she was just thirteen and my dad, the first of their eight children was born the next year.

The only land Grandpa Johnson ever owned was a cemetery plot on the hill above Belt. I think he died in 1941. I was young and unable to sit still or be quiet. I remember Grandma smacked me during the services. Carrie Johnson was buried at Highland Cemetery in Great Falls fourteen years later.

Herb, that's what everyone called my dad, except Grandma who called him Herbit when she was angry. She had a facial tic that worsened when she was upset. Her nose wiggled back and forth much like a rabbit's nose, so when she called Daddy Herbit he would wiggle his nose back at her and say, "Yes Grandma," which of course made the tic more prominent.

Dad's formal education ended with an eighth grade graduation ceremony in the tiny community of Highwood, Montana, halfway between Belt and Geraldine. Hobart Bell had homesteaded near Geraldine and my dad was not quite fifteen years old when he moved to Geraldine to work for Uncle Hobart. When the markets crashed in 1929 he agreed to stay on with his uncle for room and board.

Hobart's land was not an uncomfortable place to weather out the Great Depression. There were chickens, beef, and vegetable gardens and milk cows and the setting itself is what one would expect for a Montana ranch. Square Butte, a flat rocky mesa that sits on a lush forested base rises up behind golden wheat fields in the fall. The grassy rolling hills below Square Butte, divided by barbed wire, all belonged to my uncles. Although the sun crosses eastern flatlands in the Dakotas and collects scorching summers for Montana, when the sun falls behind the Highwoods, a range of mountain peaks that stand in a row on the western edge of the ranch, the uncomfortable heat is soon forgotten as twilight falls over the land.

While it is true that winter roars down from Canada on bitter subzero Nor'easters, and isolates ranchers, howling Chinook winds rush between mountain peaks and thaw the land temporarily bringing respite to the valley. Even today, pickups, full of cabin-fever refugees, slide through snotty gumbo to get to Geraldine for a beer and a friendly face. In 1945 I came to love my uncle's ranch and the town of Geraldine where cowboys really did exist. There I overcame fears that at age seven I could not yet put into words.

My parents met at a Grange hall dance and their courtship continued until they married in the fall of 1937.

One time my dad pointed to the restored Grand Union hotel in Fort Benton and said, "Your Mother and I were married in that building."

After their first divorce he always referred to his ex-wife as "your mother," unless he was talking to someone else, and then he called her "Carol's mother."

"Did Mother have a beautiful white dress?" I asked.

"Naw," he replied, "it wasn't really a wedding. A man came and said a few words and we signed the papers and that was all."

Then I heard him mutter to himself, "Maybe we should have had a real wedding."

My dad had a way of looking off to the left and chewing on his cheek and I knew I shouldn't ask any more questions. I was too young then to see the irony of the "Grand Union" wedding in 1937.

Daddy got a job with the WPA in 1940, (Works Progress Administration), a government program to help people get back on their feet after the Depression, and we rented a tiny house on the edge of the colored section of town. According to family legend, I was called Darlene until one afternoon when Mother was pushing me in my buggy a "nigger woman,"—a common name for black people during those years unless they were special black people who were called "Nigras"—came out of a tar papered house and screamed at her child to get away from my buggy. The little black girl's name was Darlene. .

Margaret told me Mother had taped ribbons on my bald-baby head because she hated being asked if I was a boy or a girl. That concern continued into my childhood when Daddy bought cowboy boots and Red Ryder BB guns for me. Mother tried, in spite of my bony knocked knees and red, unruly hair, to turn me into a pretty little girl. She even sewed a nylon stocking cap for me to wear at night to train my ears to lie flat. But I sucked my thumb, and as my ears flattened, my front teeth began to protrude.

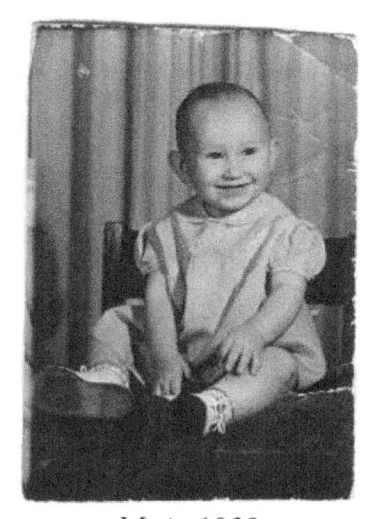

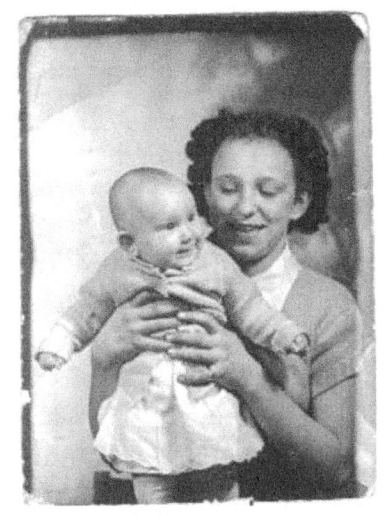

Me in 1939   with Margaret

The summer when I was three, I tried to find my way to the Davenport Hotel where Grandma Johnson still lived. Although I did arrive at the hotel's street entry, I couldn't open the heavy doors. Someone took me to the police station, and when Mother frantically called to report a lost child she was relieved to hear I was there. However, her relief had turned to anger by the time she got to the station. She found me wearing my coveralls that I had peed in and sitting on the front desk of the police station, licking on an ice cream cone. After that, Mother quit threatening to call the police if I wasn't good.

Her new threat was that she would give me to the boogie man. Nigger Joe, a very old and very black street person, pulled a wagon full of trash around town. He was a harmless fixture in the community whom most folks looked after. Sometimes Mother put leftover food on top of our garbage can for him, but I always ran and hid when I heard his wagon squeaking down our alley.

Not long after the incident at the police station I was in trouble again with my mother. I had been playing in the front yard and Mother heard water running. She glanced out the screen door and saw that I was watering the flowers; she decided I was all right. The next time she checked and I had taken off all my clothes. As she ran into the yard to pluck me from the neighbor's view, I swung around with the sprinkler just as she reached for me. Grandma Johnson joked that Mother was "mad as a wet hen." A couple of nights after that Nigger Joe came for me.

Each night I slept in my parent's bed for awhile before they moved me to the couch. I was still awake one night when I heard a knock on the door. Then I heard Mother cry, "O no! Please don't take Carol away! She'll be good. Please Joe, give her another chance."

I knew who she was talking to, and I wasn't sure that Mother would stop him from coming into the bedroom after me.

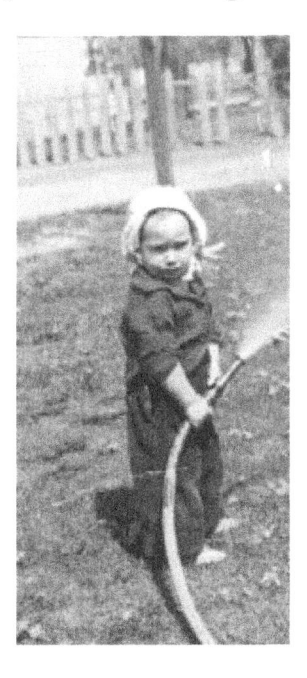

I scooted under the blankets to the foot of the bed. After a bit, I heard the door shut, and then Mother pulled me out from the bedding. She told me she made Nigger Joe go away, but I had better start being a good little girl or he might come back.

I suspect that the person at the front door was my sister who, not long after that, moved to Gardiner, Montana, to live with her brothers and her dad.

My dad had five brothers and two sisters. He was shorter than most of his brothers but when he hooked his thumbs behind his suspenders and leaned back to look past his nose they remembered he was the oldest. My dad was a bit of an enigma. His smile looked friendly, but it might be his "gotcha grin." I learned early to decipher the sincerity of the chimpanzee-like grin. Daddy liked to tease my cousins and me but sometimes he didn't stop until we were in tears.

When Daddy went to work at the Anaconda Smelter across the river in Black Eagle we moved to the west side of town and I got to know some of my cousins. Daddy's brother and his family lived in a house across the street that was built on a dry area of a slough. Uncle Toppy looked like Roy Rogers. His wife Goldie, a flamboyant bleached blonde, wore bright colors and lots of jewelry. They had three boys and a girl who all had red hair and lots of freckles, just like me. Uncle Ralph and his wife Lucille who lived on the other side of town had two girls, but only one looked like the rest of us because the other one was adopted.

The first spring after we moved to the west side the slough overflowed onto the road to Toppy's house so they all came to stay with us. I loved having other kids to play with but Mother didn't like any of Daddy's family so she was relieved when the slough receded and they moved back to their own house.

When ever Mother cooked a big Sunday dinner she invited everyone. Uncle Ralph, who had a car, brought Grandma with them. On those Sundays our house was full of noisy fun and sometimes music. Sometimes Daddy played his guitar and everyone sang or danced until late at night. But when the party lasted too long, and there was too much drinking, the fun turned into shouting and name calling.

One night, after everyone had gone home, I heard my parents arguing about how Goldie never helped with the dishes. Aunt Lucille would, if Uncle Ralph wasn't in a hurry to take Grandma home, but Goldie never even offered to help. That particular night she had too much to drink and her kids had to help her walk home. I heard Mother say, "I wish those kids would have dropped that blond hussy in the slough."

Daddy shouted back at her, "You just get off your high horse, you God damned Bo hunk. What makes you so fancy?"

Mother should have shut up when she heard Daddy use that tone of voice, but she hissed back at him: "You can't make a silk purse out of a sow's ear, and Goldie's is a pig."

I crawled under the blankets to the foot of my bed, but I could still hear Mother crying.

I loved those Sunday dinners, but when there were a lot of empty bottles on the table, the fun usually turned to fighting. All eight of Grandma's children grew up to be alcoholics. Ralph was saved at some church revival and then he quit drinking, but he got a brain tumor and died soon after his redemption. Edith quit drinking after she got out of the TB sanitarium in Oregon, but the rest of them all struggled with the disease all of their lives.

That summer Mother cleaned the chicken coop and ordered some baby chicks. One day a brown truck drove into our driveway and Mother, who assumed it was delivering the chicks she had ordered, hollered for me to come and see. The delivery man handed Mother a box with the words U.S. Army written on it. My brother Paul had joined the Army shortly after the attack on Pearl Harbor. Mother was afraid to open the box and she started to cry. Inside there was a letter and he said that he was going overseas so he was sending his things for her to keep for him.

My other brother, Walt joined the Marines, and Margaret —who got married right after she graduated—said goodbye to her new husband who was drafted into the army before their baby girl was born in the spring of 1943. Mother had a flag in her window with three blue stars because three men in her family were fighting in the war.

Margaret came to Great Falls and stayed with us while she waited for government housing and that lifted Mother's spirits. They worked side-by-side in the house, and in the garden. They laughed a lot and whispered between themselves because, "little pitchers have big ears." I loved my little niece Diane, and I watched Margaret tend to her baby so I could be a good mother to my dollies.

Everyone smoked cigarettes back then, even movie stars and school teachers. Mother and my sister frequently stopped during their household activities to have a cigarette and a cup of coffee. Daddy smoked Lucky

Strikes, which had no filter, and when I started smoking I smoked that brand too because they were there for the taking. I first tried smoking with my cousins in a cave we had dug in their yard. When I singed my hair on a candle in the cave, Mother noticed and made me tell her about our secret place. She even pried out of me the part about the boys and me taking our clothes off.

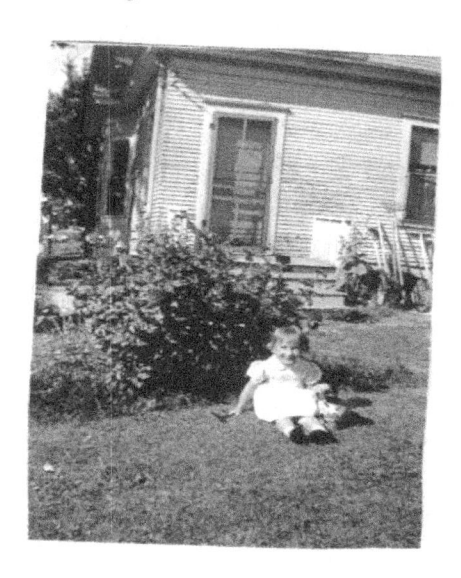

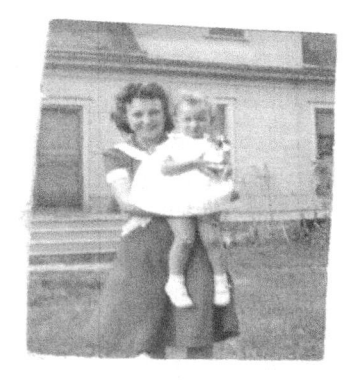

After that discovery about me and my cousins in the cave, Mother didn't cook Sunday dinners. When Uncle Ralph moved to Idaho even Grandma didn't come over anymore. Margaret moved across town into government housing, and my parents bought a house of their own out on Tenth Avenue South, so we left the Johnsons behind in the slough.

Our new house was quite large; the bedrooms were bigger than anything we had ever lived in. Mother had the basement finished into a one-bedroom apartment, and we lived there and rented the upstairs to two Airmen and their wives. Even though we lived in the basement, we lived on the right side of town, according to Mother.

Mother went to work for the Great Northern Freight House, pushing handcarts of freight from one end of a warehouse to the other. I went to a nursery school where I learned to eat the crust on three-cornered peanut butter sandwiches— because there were starving children overseas—and I learned to stay awake during nap time so I wouldn't pee in my cot.

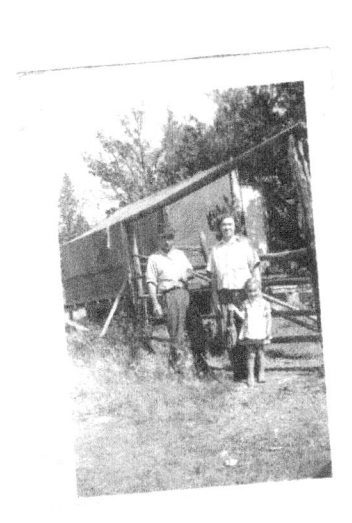

I started first grade at Emerson Grade School in 1944 and Daddy quit working at the Smelter. He took me fishing almost every day. He fished with flies that he hand-tied from old balloons and feathers, and he walked right down the middle of the rivers and streams that weren't fenced-off back then. While I looked for pretty rocks, or just sat and watched, he worked the fishing line back and forth dancing the delicate flies on clear quiet pools between shallow white water stretches. He'd pull the pole back and then snapped it onto another spot, over and over until the wicker creel that hung at his side like a purse was full of frying-pan-size trout. Sometimes when I stepped into a deep hole accidentally, Daddy would fish me out and tease me about putting me into his creel. This is a picture of me and Mother and Daddy on a weekend fishing trip.

I helped Daddy set the table and he had supper ready when Mother came home from work. If we didn't go fishing, he fried chicken and let me eat the gizzard while we waited for her. After supper Daddy usually went to town; when he came home and moved me from their bed to my roll-away bed I could smelled whiskey.

One winter night, just before Christmas, Mother woke me up and stuffed me into my snow suit. It was dark outside, and Daddy wasn't home yet. Mother told me we were going to Margaret's and when I asked why, she said she would tell me later. She yanked me out the back door and put me on my sled. As I rode on the sled through the snowy streets on that moonlight night, I wasn't sure if I should cry or not. I knew something was not right, and I was scared.

We never went back to that house. Mother filed for a divorce and we stayed at Margaret's until Mother bought another house in our same neighborhood. I stayed at the same school and had the same playmates, but everything was different and I felt shame. My nagging sense of always feeling different multiplied out of proportion during that time.

Daddy had put the deed to the big house in a poker game. I knew that my dad gambled; at least I knew as much as a six year old could know about something like that. I had gone with him sometimes to the room under the Liberty Theater. The card room was dark except for a lamp that hung over a table where men sat and smoked while they played cards. They didn't talk much, just grunted or made other noises that Daddy called bluffing. If he lost, we went home early, but if he was winning I napped on a plastic covered couch in the corner.

Mother had two more rooms built onto the one-bedroom brick house she bought. She rented the front part of the house out. We lived in the new kitchen and a bedroom and we shared the bathroom with the renters. I had to stay in the house after school each day until Mother got home from work. For awhile I was a good little girl, because I was afraid not to be.

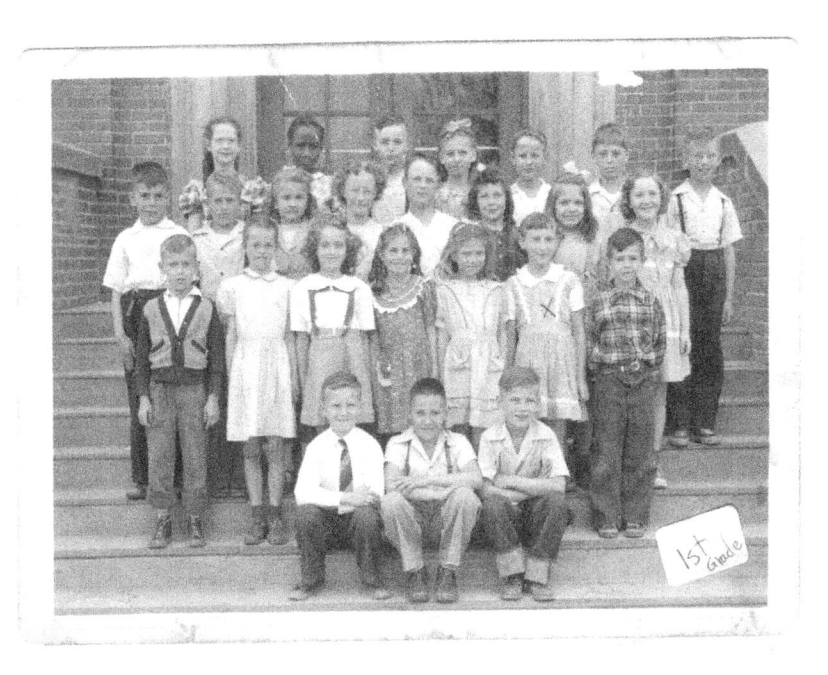

This is a picture of my first grade class at Emerson Grade school.

Some of the kids in the picture were in my class until the fifth grade. My best friend was Marlene. That's Marlene in the second row. She's on the left behind the girl with the suspenders. Marlene had blond ringlets and wore fancy dresses every day. Although she looked a little like that bratty Nelly from Little House on the Prairie, Marlene was real sweet. My boyfriend, Curtis, looked like an ad for hot dogs and baseball. We had a lot of freckles between us. He is standing next to me on the left. I was trying to hold his hand and he pulled it behind him. That's me with the Mamie Eisenhower bangs!

I thought Marlene was rich. She had her own bedroom with a picture on the wall that glowed in the dark. In her basement playroom, there was a rocking horse with real horsehair for the mane and tail, and she took piano lessons. Marlene's mother gave us fresh baked bread with butter melting on it when we came after school.

I tried to be just like Marlene. She colored carefully in one direction and her workbook always looked nice. I pressed too hard on my crayons and they broke. My workbook was a scribbled mess. I told my teacher that I had lost my workbook, and when she gave me a new one I started over from the first page, coloring as carefully as I could, but I messed that one up too.

Marlene was Mary in our Christmas program. I was a lamb. I wore a sign around my neck that said "a lamb." My parents didn't come to watch, so I didn't wave at anyone—, which our teacher told us not to do anyway, but the other kids did.

I learned to read and at first I loved the stories about Dick, Jane and Sally, but after my parent's divorce, I hated them. I wanted to live in a house with a picket fence like they did and have a daddy who went to work with a black lunch pail and a mother who wore an apron when she made homemade bread.

I was glad when first grade ended. I just wanted to go fishing with my Daddy.

CHAPTER 2—THE RODEO

The summer of 1945 was a time of conflicting events and uncertain promises both nationally and for me personally. The end of the war and the beginning of the Atomic Age were ushered in on a horrific event in Japan and the war between my parents had simmered into an exchange of civil remarks when they had to be in the same area. The first few times I went with my dad for a visit I was given spiteful messages to relay to him and he in turn supplied me with retorts to give back to my mother.

Daddy bought a small car called a coupe that summer. The trunk opened into a rumble seat where extra passengers could sit and every time Daddy came to get me, Mother made him promise not to let me ride in the rumble seat.

Daddy could go to more and better fishing holes after he bought the car and we returned to the Sun River canyon, our favorite spot many times. We also hiked up and down Wolf Creek canyon and filled his creel with pan sized trout. After we drove deep into Sheep Creek territory and walked downstream, frequently midstream, we had to walk back to the car and that meant we would need to stop at the Mountain Palace Tavern for cool drinks before heading back to Great Falls at the end of a perfect day. Some weekends we set up a tent on the banks of the Smith River that winds between precipitous canyon walls. There were no forest service regulations or private, keep-out signs. We built a fire and cooked our unlimited catch right there at our campsite. Sometimes I think it is a good thing that Daddy didn't live to see the regulations and restrictions that have made Montana off limits to regular people. Today, unless I know someone who has a place on the river, or I can afford to pay a river guide and I am willing book a couple of years in advance, I can only go to those places in my childhood memories.

When Daddy went to Uncles Hobart's to help with the harvesting he took me with him. Mother may have been concerned about horses, rattle snakes, and other dangers on a working ranch but she reluctantly agreed I could go. She packed a couple of dresses for me, just in case I needed them, but I knew cowgirls didn't wear dresses.

On the drive from Great Falls to Geraldine Daddy stopped at the Oasis Bar in Fort Benton, which was a little more than half way. Daddy said it was a watering hole made just for thirsty cowboys. He ordered a drink and bought me a soda pop. Before I finished my pop Daddy ordered another drink for himself. I worried that he would stay there drinking all day and we wouldn't get to Geraldine like he promised but we got back in the car and crossed over the Missouri river leaving the wooden boards on the bridge rattling behind us. We traveled on a gravel road that wound between fields of wheat that were beginning to turn yellow. The windows of the car were rolled down and the hot summer wind blew deliciously on my face as my excitement grew. Daddy tossed his cigarette out the window, grinned at me, and said, "Well, there it is, kiddo. That's Geraldine."

He pointed to the tall grain elevators that shimmered in the afternoon heat and explained that the mountain we could see in the background was Square Butte. Geraldine was like a proverbial one-horse town with dirt streets and wooden boardwalks. False-front buildings on each side of the street made it seem like a setting for a western movie. When we stopped at a bar called Rusty's with a saddle horse tied to a post nearby I knew we were in real cowboy country.

We walked in and a guy touched the brim of his hat and asked, "How's it going, Herb?"

"Who's your partner?" the lady behind the bar asked.

I thought Daddy must be pretty important in Geraldine. I climbed onto a bar stool and spun around a few times before he told me to stop. I had some pepperoni and a pickled egg that I got to take out of a gallon jar with a pair of tongs. The mirror on the wall behind the back bar with a huge wooden frame around it reflected the line up of colored bottles of liquor. A ceiling fan whirled overhead and spirals of yellow flypaper dotted with dead flies hung from the ceiling. Daddy had two drinks because the second one was "on the house."

"Well, are you ready to go or do you want another egg?" Daddy asked.

I was ready! We drove past the cemetery on the edge of town. I asked Daddy about a statue of a boy holding a lamb and he said a young shepard got bit by a rattlesnake. He lectured me about being careful about rattlers. I was not to pick up old pieces of metal or dig in woodpiles and I should always look on the other side of a log or a rock before I stepped over it. We passed hills and coulees with parched brown grass framed by weathered fence posts and sagging barbed wire and I felt a little frightened and a little bit excited at the same time.

Circling around the last hill I caught my first sight of Uncle Hobart's place. The faded farm house had a hedge around the yard that was brown with dust from the road. When we walked through the sagging front gate into the yard the brittle lawn crackled under our feet.

A small woman who was working with a hoe in the garden straightened up and tipped her straw hat back on her head when Daddy called to her.

"Hi," she waved as she came towards the house.

"Well, this must be little Carol!" she exclaimed. I shied behind Daddy's legs, but he pushed me into her welcoming hug. Aunt Eula was not much taller than I was, and her face looked like a wrinkled apple. Her teeth stuck out a little even when her mouth was closed, but she smiled with her eyes, and I liked that.

While Daddy and Aunt Eula looked at his new car, I looked at the buildings on the farm. The barn, red, of course, had a hay loft and there was a corral. The chicken coop and several other buildings were grey and weathered except for a steel Quonset hut that looked out of place.

Although eleven thousand homesteaders had abandoned their dream of owning a piece of Montana, the Bell boys managed to hang on through droughts and depressions and were prospering as the war was coming to an end. They were our rich relatives!

Aunt Eula showed me where the outhouse was and when I found out it was out past the garden where the rattle snakes might be lurking

I was dismayed. I hoped I would never have to go out there at night. I learned later about chamber pots.

Before I met Uncle Hobart I had a definite opinion about the longstanding debate between cattlemen and wheat growers as to which one was rightfully called a rancher. I knew Roy Rogers and Gene Autry didn't climb down from a dirty combine when the sun set in the west.

When Uncle Hobart came in for supper, I was awed by his size. He was very tall and had wide shoulders. The pearl buttons of his western shirt strained at the center and his belt buckle was almost hidden under a huge belly. When he took off his hat his white forehead showed.

"Hey," he said, "Is this our new cowhand? I do believe she is the smallest cowgirl in the state of Montana."

When he saw me shrinking under his teasing, he added, "I see she has boots. Well, I'll have to find a horse for her to ride."

Hobart and Eula had no children of their own so they eagerly welcomed their nieces and nephews into their home. The next day I met a lot of my cousins. They lived in the town of Geraldine or on nearby ranches and farms. Aunt Eula had invited everyone to come for lunch to meet me. After we got past the initial shyness they taught me how to jump out of the hayloft safely and warned me about the mean pigs. Punky, who was about my age, showed me how to gather eggs, and then we put doll clothes on the barn kittens. Uncle Hobart only had one horse that was safe enough for kids to ride, so we climbed on poor old Honey four and five at a time. By supper time the cousins and I were making lots of plans for the month ahead.

All summer, whenever any of my cousins stayed overnight, Uncle Hobart told us that whoever ate the most breakfast could be first on the horse and hold the reins. I gained weight that summer cramming down Aunt Eula's sourdough pancakes, eggs, and bacon or ham, but twelve-year-old Larry usually got to hold the reins and I had to sit behind him.

The wheat was ready to cut early in August and there wasn't much time to play. Aunt Eula cooked all the time and I set the tables and washed a lot of dishes. I went with her to the fields at noon when she took lunch to the crew. The only place to get out of the sun was under the combine, so Eula spread her feast on a tarp, and we ate with the men who took a short nap before going back to work.

If it rained hard, it was a day off and everyone headed for Geraldine. Kids joined adults in the taverns, begging for money to play the jukebox or buy candy bars. I watched Daddy deal cards at Rusty's bar, and when he took a break I stood on an orange crate behind the felt table and dealt the cards. Two for each player and me, except my last card was turned up. If anyone needed more cards, to add up to 21 points, he'd say, "Hit me," and I'd deal him another card. The guys playing cards gave me tips when Daddy came back so I never had to beg for spending money like the other kids. Late at night, sleepy kids, dogs and drunken cowboys were loaded into muddy pickups for the drive back to their ranches.

One day I overheard Uncle Hobart and my dad talking about a rodeo in Geraldine. The men who waited in line with their trucks full of grain at the elevators were talking about a rodeo too. In fact most of the town was talking about a rodeo and they were saying there would be a parade, a greased pig race and even fireworks. It was true! Geraldine was going to have its first rodeo and my uncle was named the grand marshal. Daddy asked me what I thought about riding a yearling steer in the rodeo. He said he would talk with Uncle Hobart about it if I wanted to try it. I would be the youngest rider and I liked the idea right away, but Aunt Eula didn't. She reminded Daddy he would have to answer to my mother if I got hurt. Uncle Hobart promised he would at least think about it. I told my cousins that I was going to ride in the rodeo and they wanted to ride too so we tried to practice on the milk cow. She just ambled to the barn with one of us on board.

All of my aunts said "no way" to any rodeoing for their kids, but Uncle Hobart decided to let me enter the rodeo as a rider. Daddy put a loud speaker on one of the farm trucks and drove around town announcing, "The youngest cowgirl in Montana will be riding in the Geraldine rodeo on Labor Day."

Between harvesting and partying, the ranchers in the area found time to build bleachers around an area that they plowed and smoothed into a soft surface for the upcoming show. They built chutes out of lodge pole pine so the riders could climb down the poles, straddle the animal and get a good hold before giving a signal to open the gate.

Daddy bought me a white cowboy hat, a real one without the string that goes under your chin. I tied a large hankie around my neck and Uncle Hobart borrowed a fancy saddle for Honey.

I knew that Daddy had to take me back to Great Falls the day after the rodeo so I could start second grade and I tried not to cry while I packed my suitcase but I didn't want to go back. I wanted to stay in Geraldine with Uncle Hobart and Aunt Eula forever. I reasoned that they didn't have any kids and they would like to have a little girl. My mother worked all the time and I figured I could visit her sometimes. I didn't ask Daddy or my aunt and uncle if I could stay but I prayed and wished on the first star each evening.

Labor Day morning came. I was pretty puffed up with my own importance as I rode on Honey behind my uncles who led the parade on horseback. They carried the American flag and the Montana state flag. I waved my hat to the people lined up on the boardwalks and they waved back, especially my cousins.

I was scheduled to be the third rider and while I waited my turn I stood on the poles of the chutes and watched the yearling steer paw at the dirt. When it was time, I climbed down the poles and placed my legs around the frightened animal. I felt his muscles quiver. A cowboy told me I could use both hands, but I wanted to do it right so I grabbed onto the hard metal of the sirsingle with my left hand and raised my right arm into the air.

I heard my Dad announce, "Ladies and Gentlemen, turn your attention to chute number two. Seven-year-old Carol Johnson, the youngest cowgirl in the State of Montana will be riding Dynamite!"

"Are you ready?" the cowboy asked.

I nodded, and he opened the gate. Dynamite hesitated a minute, then ran straight into the center of the arena. I remember thinking, "Shoot, this is easy." Then the steer turned inside out and I was in the air. The crowd was very quiet until I finally got up and waved my hat, like Daddy had told me to. Then there was a loud roar from the bleachers. I don't remember hitting the ground, and for that matter, I don't remember much that happened that afternoon.

I woke up while I was resting in the back seat of the car, and a cowboy was talking to me through the window. He gave me a jackknife with his name engraved on it and I learned later that he was a champion rodeo rider. Other people came by to see if I was all right, and I must have looked like I was, but my head hurt and I felt like throwing up.

In the evening, before the dance and the fireworks that I missed—along with the greased pig race that I had wanted to enter—I went with Daddy to Rusty's bar. Someone had put a jar out to collect donations for me because I hadn't won any prizes at the rodeo. I felt dizzy and went outside to sit on the boardwalk in the cool air. As I sat there holding my head, I heard someone say, "Mommy, look, there's the youngest cowgirl in Montana." The little boy was hiding behind his mom and sneaking looks at me as they came across the street.

Daddy put me on Honey and she found her way home without my help. I rode the mile and a half back to the ranch with my face in the horse's sweet smelling mane. Daddy and I agreed that we would wait awhile before telling Mother about the rodeo.

I was a very small seven-year-old the summer of my rodeo debut. I don't think I would have wanted any of my children to do the same thing, but the rodeo was the highlight of my childhood. It changed how I felt about being different. From that summer on, I was different in a special way.

CHAPTER 3—PEACETIME

My second grade classmates at Emerson grade school were not impressed with my story about riding a wild steer in a rodeo. In fact, Marlene, with her hands on her hips, stuck her face in mine and called me a liar. She said she was going to ask my mom if I really did ride in a rodeo. Of course, when I told her my mother didn't know about it she was sure I had made up the whole story. Roger and Leroy may have believed me, but Roger said, "So what! Anyone can ride a baby cow." I had experienced something wonderful and unique but the thrill of the adventure was diluted as I shared my excitement.

The war was over in the fall of 1945 and our country was in a celebrating mood. The truce that my parents had agreed on ended when Mother saw some home movies of the rodeo. My dad's friend had filmed the rodeo, and he invited a few people to gather in the basement of the downtown establishment to see his pictures. I was happy about my Mother and Dad being together and I was as surprised as my mother was when I saw myself in the middle of the screen riding Dynamite. My hat flew off and my legs flopped up and down. Then I went head first onto the ground. Mother jumped out of her chair, and started yelling and cussing at Daddy, right in front of the other people"Damn it, Herb," she screamed. "What the hell were you thinking? She could have been killed!"

Mother dragged me like a rag doll up the stairs, past the customers on their barstools, and out the door, leaving Daddy to deal with the people in the basement who had witnessed Mother's wrath.

The next day I heard Mother talking to Margaret on the phone. She said my dad just used me to get attention. She complained that he was a dreamer, and he put those ideas into my head too. She told Margaret that I was already talking about riding in the Augusta rodeo next year.

"You know how wild that whole town is that week. A little girl has no business being around all those drunken cowboys."

Mother didn't talk to Daddy when he picked me up the next weekend to go fishing, but when we came back she had calmed down and offered him a cup of coffee. She may have been right about Daddy enjoying the attention he got because of his little cowgirl, but she was definitely right about my dreams. I was ready for the next rodeo. Most of all, I wanted a horse of my own. I wished on the first star each night for one. Every morning I checked the yard to see if my wish came true.

Actually, a horse did come into our back yard one time, but not because of a wishing star. An old, shaggy Shetland pony roamed free around our neighborhood and everyone made sure the orphaned horse had water, carrots, apples and other scraps. He was no Trigger or Champion but he was good enough for me. The day he showed up in our yard I gave him a couple of sugar cubes and tied him to our picket fence. I didn't say any prayers that night or wish on any stars. I took one last look at my shaggy horse before I pulled the shade down on the window in the kitchen, and hoped Mother wouldn't look in the yard. The next morning he was gone, and so was part of the fence. Mother spanked me and told me I had to stop the horse nonsense.

I really got into trouble when I went for a horseback ride with a strange man. He wasn't a stranger to me because he came to the water pump near our house every week and I made sure I was there to pet the horses that pulled his wagon. Sometimes he let me sit on a horse. One day he unhooked the trailer, put me on one of the horses, and got on behind me. When we rode by my house, I saw Mother outside in the garden; I waved and shouted happily. She ran toward us cussing and screaming, and yanked me off the horse. She told me to get into the house, and kept screaming at the man. When she came in I tried to tell her he was my friend, a real nice man, but she spanked me with a belt that time.

It seemed that Mother never believed me. She always listened to the other story. One time the boys in the neighborhood built a fort; and I wanted to see inside. They agreed to let me in if I would show them something. I was in the clubhouse before I figured out that what they wanted to see was all of me, and I couldn't go back on my word. I was more ashamed that the boys had tricked me than I was about showing them my girl part. But the incident bothered me a lot, and I made the mistake of confiding in Mother. She called the oldest boy and when she asked him what had happened, he said I told them they needed to let me in their clubhouse because I had something to show them. After he left, I cried and pleaded with Mother to believe me, but she spanked me hard.

Another time, one of the kids in the neighborhood called me a "fucker" and I had him on the ground and was whaling on his face with my fists when Mother pulled me off. She shook me hard and told me to stop fighting with the boys. "What kind of a little girl are you?" she scolded. When I tried to tell her what the boy had called me, thinking that she would say he needed a good beating, she refused to listen to what I was trying to say except for the "f" word, which she heard loud and clear. For that, she shoved a bar of soap into my mouth, and rubbed it around on my teeth. What I learned from her harsh discipline was to keep everything to myself, and not get caught.

When Daddy and I visited Geraldine that fall, I asked Aunt Eula if I could sleep on the cot on the sun porch instead of with my dad. She didn't ask why and I was glad I didn't have to tell that Daddy touched me "down there" sometimes.

One weekend while we were at Geraldine, Daddy and I went to a turkey shoot. We didn't shoot turkeys. It was a contest to see who could hit closest to the bull's eye on a paper target. The best shot won a turkey. I entered the kid's division, and somehow shot better than my country cousins. The first place prize for kids was a beautiful white goose. Daddy made a cage for my goose in the back yard, and I put a sign on my playhouse that said, "The White Goose Club." The neighbor kids were excited to join my club. We met twice a week, and had a password and other secrets that only grade school kids would know. I was the president and I took roll call. The penalty for missing a meeting was providing snacks for the next meeting.

School let out early the Wednesday before Thanksgiving, and I raced out of Emerson along with my classmates, excited about our four-day vacation. Mother wasn't home when I got there, and when I went out to the clubhouse the goose was gone! As soon as I saw the car, I ran to the driveway crying that my goose was gone. Mother held me by each shoulder, and squatting down to my level said, "I knew you would be mad, but I took the goose to the butcher. He is going to be our Thanksgiving bird."

I pulled away from her and started to run, but then I stopped and turned to look at her in disbelief. I tried to breathe without crying. I couldn't believe she had done that. I ran into the house before she could see my tears.

On our way to Margaret's the next day, Mother told me I should be proud that I provided a nice bird for the family's Thanksgiving dinner.

"Besides, I didn't like all those secret meetings you and your friends were having out in that shed."

I pouted, and refused to come to the table where my goose, the centerpiece, was cooked to perfection by Mother. She kept adding comments like, "Surely you are old enough to know we can't keep a goose in the city limits." She just didn't understand that not only was my goose dead, but I wasn't the president of The White Goose Club anymore.

That November families across the United States were gathering around their Thanksgiving tables with special reason. Many chairs that had been empty on previous holidays were filled by servicemen who had made it home safely. For those unfortunate families with chairs that would always remain empty, there was the thanks that the nightmare was over and that their sons had not died in vain. That day, my sister's husband was at our table to carve my goose, and although Mother's oldest son was wounded in Iowa Jima, he did recover.

Daddy stayed overnight with us on Christmas Eve. In the morning, he drove to town to get Grandma Johnson. Uncle Toppy, Aunt Goldie and my cousins came for dinner too. Mother cooked a turkey and I was done pouting about the goose. The grownups sat at the small table in the kitchen, but my cousins and I sat on the bed balancing paper plates full of turkey and pumpkin pie while listening to the radio.

Right before school started in January, Mother got a phone call from someone in Roundup. Her dad was in the hospital, and her mother had been arrested. I wasn't close to my grandparents in Roundup. They didn't speak English and they didn't even look American. Grandmother wore long bulky dresses with multicolored aprons, and a scarf on her head that she tied between her double chins. Her face was very round, and deeply wrinkled like an Appalachian apple doll. Some of her teeth were gone, which made her top lip suck back into her mouth sometimes. Grandpa was a tiny man, and very thin. He wore suspenders to hold up oversized wool trousers. With a head of wild wiry hair and a bushy moustache, he looked like Albert Einstein. He had the final say in their home, but he did step aside when Grandma was at the cook stove. After his day in the coal mine, he put his head under the spigot outside and pumped well water over his head until it ran clear. Then he dried off with old gunnysacks; still soot stayed in the creases of his skin and around his eyes.

Home to my grandparents was a one-room company house. A feather bed was hidden by a curtain hung across the end of the room. When I see pictures of angels lying around on fluffy clouds, I think of how wonderful that bed felt. I sank deep into its softness, and drifted off to sleep to the drone of a strange language. Grandma cooked on a woodstove; she pumped water from the well in the yard, and used an outhouse. She kept chickens and goats that she milked. She made cheese from the goat's milk, but limburger cheese was always a pungent staple in their tiny house.

When Mother and I stepped off the Greyhound bus in Roundup, it was beginning to snow. We trudged down the dimly lit sidewalk carrying our suitcases. The front door to the small hospital was locked but a nurse with a hat that looked like it was made out of white cardboard, and who had a million keys hanging on her belt, unlocked the door. Grandpa was propped up on several pillows. He didn't have a shirt on, and his left shoulder was wrapped in bandages. He was cleaner than I had remembered him, and there was color in his cheeks. He told Mother the doctor said he could go home in a couple of days. They talked in Czech, and we left after Mother gave Grandpa a kiss on his clean cheek. While we were walking from the hospital to the jail, Mother told me that Grandma had accidentally shot Grandpa with the shotgun they kept by the stove.

At the Musselshell County jail, we had to leave our suitcases in the office; the sheriff made us take our coats off too. Then he took us in the back where grandmother was sitting on a cot in a cell, staring at her hands resting on the shelf of her belly. When she saw us she began rocking back and forth and moaning. Mother reached through the bars toward Grandma, and when Grandma came close they hugged and kissed between the bars. At first they both were crying, and then they started talking at the same time and began to laugh. When I was older, I learned what had really happened that winter night. Grandpa had been gone for two days and two nights, chasing women and drinking; when he came home drunk the second night Grandma shot him. The neighbors called the police after Grandpa ran into the street screaming. He didn't press charges, and we brought him home from the hospital the day after Grandma was released.

In the spring I came down with the chickenpox and Grandma Johnson stayed with me while Mother was working. One afternoon my mother and dad called to say they were in Missoula and that they had gotten married again. I wasn't sure what that meant for all of us, and I wasn't sure how to feel about it, but I pretended to be happy because they sounded like they were. I guessed Daddy would live with us again; and I wondered where he was going to sleep. I also wondered if there would be any more summer trips to Geraldine. Mother brought home a rollaway bed from Missoula and I slept in the kitchen after that.

Margaret had a baby boy in July so Diane stayed with us for two weeks. She had thick brown hair that Mother weaved into long braids. I thought she was the cutest niece a girl could have. We played dolls under the row of cottonwoods in my back yard, and ran through the sprinkler on hot afternoons. Mother's family was growing. My brothers had children too, but to me our real family was just the three of us. I was a Johnson and everyone else was a Pollock. I guess Mother was both.

I knew Daddy was drinking whiskey again because I could smell it when he tucked me in. Some Saturdays I went with him as he made his rounds to downtown bars and taverns. When Daddy said he was going to town, he didn't mean he was going to Woolworths or Newberys. He went to the first two blocks of Central where the Glenwood Bar and

Hussman's Pool Parlor were. Then he crossed the street to the Mint Bar where original paintings by Charlie Russell once hung. Daddy had been in the Mint one time when the now famous western artist was there, but Daddy never really met Kid Russell.

In the back room of the Mint, men sat and waited for results of horse races to be posted on a large blackboard. They placed bets on their favorite horse at a barred window, like the booth at the movie theater. The room was so thick with cigarette smoke that I could hardly see across it. In the Club Cigar Store, a door opened into the alley, which was part of skid row. Daddy and I stepped over broken wine bottles, and occasionally broken winos sleeping off yet another cheap drunk, as we made our way to First avenue south, the official skid row in Great Falls.

The buildings were not that much different from those on Central avenue. The doors had a couple of rectangular windows to peep through so a person could see if any one he knew, or didn't want to know, was sitting at the long bars. Barstools and foot rails provided some respite for the weary travelers who staggered from place to place in search of a free drink. Above street level were rooms, apartments and flop houses. When worn-out drunks and addicts hit bottom, they moved to skid row, and some of them died there. There were no "hello, my name is" places back then. Teddy, my dad's youngest brother spent his time and money on skid row whenever he came to town from the sheep camps where he sobered up. Teddy had killed a man in a drunken brawl when he was younger and spent some time in the Montana State Prison. Daddy showed me where the fight had taken place, and where the man had hit his head on the curb. When Teddy could get away from the isolated existence he had chosen, he came to town and shared his paychecks. When he arrived, he treated his cronies to good whiskey, but after a few days they had to resort to drinking Canned Heat in the alley, and when that was gone it was time for Teddy to go back to the sheep. Daddy told me Teddy purposely got thrown in jail for public drunkenness during the holidays because the meals at the jail were good, and the jail always gave gifts of socks or tobacco.

The working ladies in the upstairs rooms on skid row were nice to me. They bought me soda pop and other treats. They wore beautiful bright-colored silk clothes and very high-heeled shoes. I thought they were beautiful, and I was proud that they all knew my dad. There were slot machines and punch boards in some of the bars and Daddy paid the bartender so I could push the plug of paper through the hole in the punch board and then unravel the paper to see if I won. Sometimes I did win a free soda pop or a bag of smoked salmon, but I never won the big teddy bears that hung behind the bar. When I put a nickel in a slot machine and pulled the handle, I held my breath while I waited for lemons or cherries to line up in a row. When they did, a few nickels came out the bottom of the machine. I liked going to town with Daddy, but I didn't talk about those downtown trips with Mother.

There was something else I didn't talk to Mother about. When Margaret asked me if Daddy ever touched me "funny," I pretended I didn't know what she meant. She told me he should never touch me "down there," even during my bath, and to be sure and tell her or Mother if he did.

Mother loved the State Fair. I did too. In 1947 Gene Autry came to the fair with his palomino horse, Champion. He led the parade down Central Avenue and across the bridge to the main gate where he cut the ribbons on opening day. I ran alongside the parade all the way to the stone gates of the fairgrounds. Mother and I went to the fair every day for the whole week. We walked through the livestock barns and exhibits in the mornings while the buildings were cool, and after eating a picnic lunch she had packed, we lay under the cottonwoods and rested until the horse races and rodeo began. That year we had matching outfits. Our western shirts had flowers embroidered across the front and down the sleeves, and the slacks had the same design on the front pockets. Following the events at the grandstand, we played bingo and sometimes ate corn-on-the cob cooked on a stick. With a cup of hot butter to dip the corn in, we tried not to get our outfits dirty. The biggest mess, of course, was cotton candy, but it was worth every sticky problem. Mother rode some of the carnival rides, and although I was afraid to ride the Ferris wheel, I did.

My friend Billy Accord died. He wasn't sick and he didn't have an accident; he just died. We were nine years old and in the fourth grade. On the day that Billy died, I rode my bike over to Dorothy and Barbara's house to see if they wanted to go bike riding. They were two of Billy's many cousins that lived on our same block. The girls were sitting on their porch when I screeched to a stop in their driveway spraying gravel against their house. They said "hi," kind of quiet, and told me they couldn't play. When I asked why, they said they weren't supposed to talk about it. Then their Mother came to the screen door and told me to run along. I figured she was mad about the gravel. As I was pushing my bike down the alley, Bertha's mother came out to empty her garbage. When she saw me she said she sure was sorry about my little friend Billy. She looked at me kind of funny, and then she said, "You do know that Billy died, don't you?"

I didn't answer her. My heart was racing a mile a minute, and I ran the rest of the way to my house. The screen door banged behind me, and Mother shouted at me to stop slamming the door. I spit out my news, "Guess what! Billy Accord died."

Mother grabbed me by my shoulders and shook me hard. "Don't ever, ever make a joke about something like that," she said.

I started to cry, and then the phone rang. After Mother hung up, she looked at me and started to cry.

"My God," she said, "I just gave him a ride home from school the other day."

Mother sat at the table with her head in her hands and sobbed while I stood behind her and patted her back. I thought it was strange that she was so sad about Billy, because she didn't really know him or his family.

When we heard that he had been playing tag with some other kids, and he just fell down on the ground and died, it made death seem so possible for all of us. There would be other "Billy" type deaths in later years and as a medical person I would understand the sudden cardiac accident that killed my friend, but the unexplained death at that time left the doors to the darkest parts of my imagination open. They would not close for many years.

Croxford's mortuary is a Gothic-like structure with spires and gargoyles. An ornate brick pattern surrounds the wooden castle-like double door entrance. The hearse, a long black limousine, is parked under a cloth awning in front of double glass doors. After funerals, the coffin is rolled out through those doors and into the hearse for the trip to the cemetery. On the day of Billy's funeral, the red-carpeted church-like mortuary was full of our friends from Emerson. Everyone was dressed in their Sunday school clothes, and their parents were there too. Billy lay in a white coffin up at the front of the church with his Sunday school suit on. His family sat behind a curtain on one side of the room up front; I could hear them crying. A preacher said some prayers, and a lady behind another curtain sang some of the church songs that I knew. One of the songs was "rocketages." The preacher said what a lucky little boy Billy was to get to be with Jesus so soon, and then everyone walked up to look at Billy in the coffin. Mother walked too fast so I didn't get a good look, but I waved goodbye. At Highland Cemetery, just blocks from where Billy and I had played every day, his coffin was lowered into a hole in the ground. His mother screamed, and her family had to drag her to back to the car. Her screams echoed across the prairie that day and across my memory for many years.

In the spring of 1948, Mother went to a place called the Mayo Clinic. I didn't know why, and when I asked I was told it was grownup stuff and not to worry about it. After that she went on another trip to an Oral Robert's revival, but I didn't care about that much because it was in the summer and I got to go to Geraldine. Like children do, I sensed the changes in our daily lives could be ominous. Mother didn't work after I turned ten in July. Daddy bought a wooden trailer house with a bed and a stove in it. He pulled it up to the Sun River canyon and claimed a spot. The three of us stayed under the shadow of Sawtooth Mountain the rest of the summer. While Daddy and I hiked around the mountainside or watched the Sun River crash over boulders and rush through rock crevices, Mother picked wildflowers and took naps in a chair at the campsite. At night, under more stars than the three of us could count, we roasted marshmallows or sang while Daddy played the guitar. Summer ended. I learned about something called cancer. I wasn't supposed to talk about it with any of my friends. In 1948 people with cancer were shunned and feared, and because Mother had "female cancer" the disgrace was multiplied.

I started fifth grade. Mother started going to a Holy Roller church and Daddy moved to town to live with his mother. I walked to town on weekends to see Daddy and Grandma, and I went to the movies or with Daddy on his rounds to the bars and skid row.

My parents got divorced again, but that time I didn't care if my friends knew about it, as long as they didn't know my mother had cancer.

Mother went to the hospital a lot that fall, and when she was in the hospital I stayed at Margaret's so I could walk to school. I liked living with my sister and being an auntie to Diane and Gary. They had routines in their home. Each day after supper, we had time to play before we took our baths, and then Margaret gave us a snack and listened to our prayers. We all had to go to bed at 8 p.m. The predictability felt good in a strange way, and I began to look forward to Mother's trips to the hospital.

Before Christmas, Mother and I moved to the Brent Hotel, a tenement apartment not far from skid row. I didn't know we were going to move until the house was sold. I came home from school one day and saw our car packed full of stuff, even our ironing board. I cried when we drove away, and Mother did too. We set up housekeeping in one room with a double bed, a dresser and a small sink in the corner. We cooked on a hotplate, and shared the showers and toilets down the hall with the other people in the building. Two narrow and very tall windows in our room faced a small grocery store across the street. A bar with a flashing neon light was next to the grocery store; and even when we pulled the window shades down, we could see the light flashing on and off until the middle of the night.

The Brent was over a mile from Emerson grade school; we were out of that district. Mother said I could keep going to Emerson, but I would have to walk farther. She cautioned me not to tell anyone we had moved. When school started in January, I walked to Emerson every morning and lived in my old life. After school I left the world that I had lost, and walked through new neighborhoods to the unknown reality of the Brent Hotel. I passed one week in that limbo before I blurted out my misery to a favorite teacher. I had to move to another school district.

CHAPTER 4—THE MAKING OF AN ORPHAN

Mother put up a miserable little Christmas tree on our dresser. It was a fake one, so we left the lights on all night. We went to Margaret's for Christmas Eve, and Mother let me drink a small glass of 7-up and Mogan David wine. Christmas morning we opened the gifts and then we walked to the Greyhound Bus Depot. I carried my new doll and a suitcase of doll clothes to play with on the long ride to Roundup.

The bus traveled along silvery roads winding through snow berms separating the ribbon of road from the endless snow-covered land. I looked through bridge trestles at banks of fog that crept along the river beds frosting remnants of summer past.

My grandparents' little house looked like an igloo with only the door showing, but a warm fire in the cook stove welcomed us. We ate potato latkes with homemade applesauce and sour cream, as Mother and Grandma chattered away in their native tongue. We stayed just one night. When we returned to the bus station the next day to continue our trip to see Paul in Livingston, Mother and Grandmother wept in each other's arms. Margaret told me one time that Mother never believed she would die. I wonder about that when I think back to that Christmas trip across Montana in the dead of winter. After a poignant visit with my brothers and their families, we came back to Great Falls in time for me to start a new school.

At Largent elementary school I discovered the wonderful world of hot lunches. Meals cooked in the basement during spelling class each morning sent aromas up to the third floor. The cafeteria-style meal, with as many helpings as I wanted, wasn't TV-tray bits and pieces like my grandchildren get at school now. We were offered three or four different items, or a large portion of stew with dumplings, or real macaroni and cheese, baked till the cheese strung across the pan when it was served. We even had fried chicken sometimes. Some days, that noon meal was all I had.

That winter I discovered—-and have continued to believe— that fifth grade boys are the nastiest and meanest bunch of creeps alive. At Largent, Lonnie was the leader of that vile gang. When the teacher left the room, he and his followers stood at their desks and jerked their third finger up and down at her departure. Not only was Lonnie the leader of the boys, he was also the blond, blue eyed darling all the girls swooned over. One Friday when I was staying with Margaret, he called and asked me to meet him in the balcony of the Liberty Theater on Saturday morning. "O, God, I've just got to go!" I begged my sister. My first mistake was using God's name, not allowed in their home. Margaret said Mother would never allow me to meet a boy at the movies. My sister not only said no, but grounded me to the bedroom that evening with no snack. I was really mad at Margaret for not letting me go to the movie. I had tried really hard to fit into her family, but there were so many rules. That time, I was glad she said no to me, because when I returned to school on Monday, I learned that all but three girls in our class—and thanks to my too strict sister I was one of them— had gone to the balcony to meet Lonnie where his gang sat giggling from the back row.

I played a secret game that spring; rich in symbolism I wasn't aware of then. While I was rummaging through handouts at the Salvation Army, I found a blue satin skirt that I fashioned into a cape. With a few other items, I became Supergirl. I hid the outfit in a closet on the second floor of the hotel; after school I sneaked upstairs to become a powerful, magical hero who slunk around the hotel halls looking for evil to overthrow.

The Salvation Army was just across the street from our new home, so were the police and fire station. I had way too much free time on my hands while Mother, probably drugged with pain medication, slept. The firemen took me in like a mascot. I quickly figured out they cooked their supper at 5:30 each day; they put a plate on the table for me. In the back room, where they restored old or broken toys donated for their Christmas drive I spent many afternoons sanding and painting wooden parts. I felt proud to be helping the poor. I also spent a lot of time hanging around the city jail. I visited the prisoners, probably serving time for petty crimes or public drunkenness like Uncle Teddy, through barred windows.

The Salvation Army ladies served a nice supper after their evening church services. It was free but Mother was not happy about my hanging around the winos and other down-and-outers. She said we had money, and if I was hungry I could go to the lunch counter at the bus station.

We did have money; Mother was very resourceful. When she sold our house, she invested in stamp machines, which she placed around town. After she became bedridden, the maintenance of the stamp machines fell on me. My rounds, which I made on my bicycle, began at The First National Bank. I cashed Mother's check and put the cash into a bank bag that went into my Roy Rogers lunch pail for disguise. The U.S. Post Office was my next stop, and there I purchased rolls of stamps for the machines. At each stop, I opened the stamp machine with a key, inserted a roll of stamps, and removed money from the machine. The last stop was at the bank again, where I emptied the Roy Rogers safe and got a deposit slip for Mother's records. I also did other banking and errands for Mother, and began to understand the role money played in our security.

But another thing I learned about was credit. Mother had set up a charge account at the corner grocery. And Mr. Harvey was aware that I did the shopping for Mother and me. When I came home one fateful day, Mother was propped against the pillows in her bed with the grocery bill in front of her. She told me that Mr. Harvey had taken advantage of me and was cheating us. She said our bill for the last month was way too high, and she was going to call him and get to the bottom of it! O boy, I thought, this is it; I'm really in trouble now. As she reached for the telephone, I confessed to charging some candy and soda pop. As I've said before, my mother never took my side in any situation, but she said there was no way a child could run up a bill that high. I had been treating a lot of kids at school, but I didn't argue any more as she lit into Mr. Harvey on the phone. He knocked off part of the bill, and asked Mother to sign each shopping list she sent with me in the future. I suppose he felt sorry for Mother, but I could tell by that way he treated me after that that he didn't feel sorry for me. After that I just stole change out of the glass chicken Mother kept on top of the medicine chest.

I would have been a challenge to any middle-aged mother but, given the circumstances, my Mother had little or no control over me. I stole a huge beach ball from the dime store one time, and when Mother found it in our closet with the price tag still on it, she made me inflate it and carry it back to the store. I ditched it in a garbage can in an alley, and lied about what the clerk at the store said. No doubt Mother's anger was inflamed by her pain and immobility, but although I learned to dodge flying coffee cups, I couldn't ignore the cruel words she flung at me as she raged from her bed. I cried and run to the toilet room down the hall and locked myself inside a stall. Hidden behind the door, I would stuff my fists into my eyes and pray that she would die.

Mother was doing her own praying. I came home from school one day and saw several ladies kneeling at the foot of her bed. They were swaying and modulating their words in unison as Mother bent her chin to her chest. One of the woman motioned for me to join them on my knees, which I did, but when Mother looked at me I had to bite my cheeks so I wouldn't smile. Those women were jabbering in different languages and moaning. I didn't know whether to laugh or to go into the hall to get my Supergirl outfit. Later, Margaret said she was not happy about the Holy Roller ladies visiting Mother, because she thought they were trying to get Mother to leave her money to their church when she died. I was surprised that my sister talked to me about such a grown up thing, but I felt justified in refusing to kneel with them the next time they visited.

My dad was out of the picture during this time. Grandma Johnson told me that he had forced himself on my Mother in her horrible condition. I hated my mind's picture of that story. One of the other things I hated was putting Mother's bloody sanitary pads in the garbage. Mother handed me the pads and I had to wrap them in newspaper. I knew there was blood, and I thought there were sores inside her. I didn't want to think about my dad doing something so ugly! So I chose not to believe it and as I got older I wondered why my Grandma would tell a child something like that even if it were true.

I began faking headaches so I could stay home. I was afraid of what might happen during the day when Mother was all alone. Mother misinterpreted my complaints as signs that I might be coming into my womanhood. She explained that as my body changed and I became a young lady I would bleed, like she did, each month, and that I would have to wear a sanitary pad. I heard "blood" and "pads," and equated that with her blood and pads! God, how I dreaded my monthly "visits."

I wondered what would happen to me if Mother did die. I assumed I would live with Margaret, and I was anxious to get on with that part of my life. Mother had some good days that last summer. We picnicked at Giant Springs with Margaret' family. When she was up to it, Mother went dancing with her girl friend Kelly who was divorced, and had three kids. They lived at St. Thomas Orphanage. Once a month the kids got to come home for a weekend. I became friends with them when our Mothers dropped us off at Mitchell pool or Gibson Park while they shopped or just sat in the car visiting. They told me they liked living at St. Thomas because they got to do a lot of things free, like going to rodeos and the fair and all the parades. I told Mother I wished I could go to their school, and I am sure she was relieved to hear that as she had already arranged for me to visit the school. On the Fourth of July the school attended a rodeo at the fairgrounds, and I was invited to go too. The orphans sat together in the grandstand, and when the announcer asked the crowd to welcome the kids from St. Thomas, I yelled as loud as the others. It felt good to be part of a gang. When the St. Thomas bus stopped to let me off at the Brent we had finished singing about one hundred bottles of beer on a wall and I knew I wanted to go to school at St. Thomas. Mother made arrangements for me to enter the orphanage in September and Margaret helped her shop for the navy blue uniforms I would need.

Mother was in and out of the hospital many times that summer and I stayed with my sister. Each morning my niece and I counted how many of the morning glories climbing past Margaret's kitchen window had opened before we set up our dollhouses in the grass.

Sometimes Margaret would give us some blankets to pin over the clothesline to make a stage and we would put on a play for the kids in the neighborhood. On shopping days we rode the bus downtown with my sister. We all dressed up in our nicest clothes and wore hats and gloves. On the best days we stopped at Woolworth's soda fountain.

In my heart and on the palm of my right hand I carry the scars from that summer. I had a large wart on my hand that bled when I picked at it. Mother was undergoing radiation treatment so she took me to the Great Falls Clinic where the nurse placed my hand under a long tube and radiated my wart. It disappeared except for a faint discoloration. The scar in my heart is not faint. Life twists around, and my experiences have enabled me to examine old wounds from a different perspective. I returned to the same clinic for my own course of radiation treatment in later years and I found my mother's fear, terror, courage and resignation.

There were no trips to the Montana State Fair that year. Mother was admitted to the hospital for the last time in August.

Margaret took me to the hospital to see Mother. I was told to be as quite as a mouse because children were not allowed in the hospital. After dark, her husband drove us around the back of the building and when no one was looking we slipped through the door, and crept up three flights of gray marbled stairs. We tiptoed across the hall to a room where Mother, who was lost in bedding of her same pale color, was propped against several pillows. She looked very small and her eyes were sunk deep into her face. When she spoke, her voice was scratchy; and I could hardly hear her. She said,

"I love you Carol, you be a good girl."

She stared at me for a long time like she was trying to memorize how I looked. She didn't cry; I didn't either as, I waved goodbye when we left the room.

Two weeks later, I woke up in my sister's bed instead of on her couch where I had fallen asleep. I could hear Diane and Gary at the breakfast table, and wondered why I was in bed. My sister was sitting on the side of the bed, and her face was all puffy. Tears from her red eyes ran down her cheeks, and I knew what she was going to say. "Mother died last night. Breakfast is ready, but you can stay here as long as you need to."

I felt like I was in a play. Margaret had just spoken her part, and I didn't know my lines because we hadn't rehearsed the scene. I didn't feel like crying, but I thought I should. I knew I shouldn't smile when I went out to the table, but I was afraid I might. I lay there for what I thought might be an appropriate amount of time. When I was sure I could keep a sad face on, I went to the breakfast table. Throughout the next few days I searched for clues from others that would show me how to act. I had no feelings of my own to act upon.

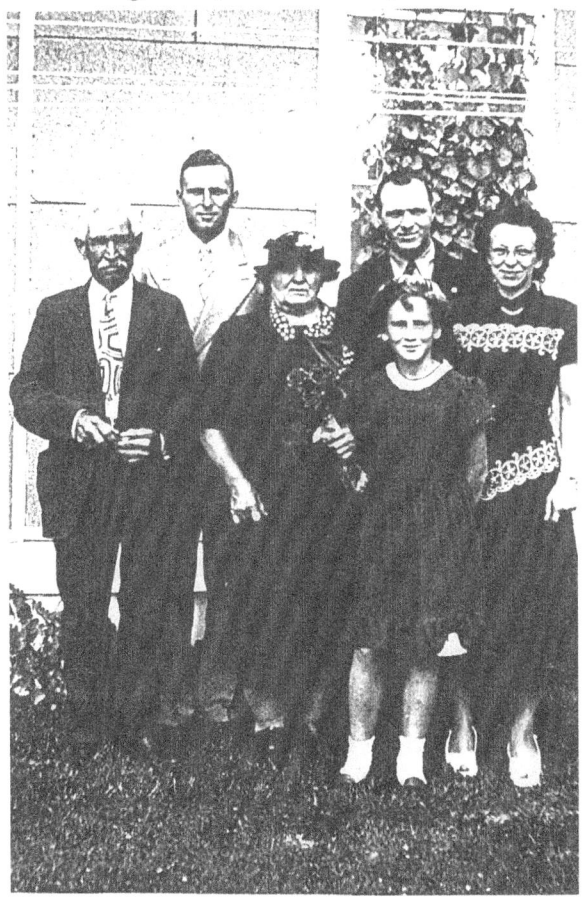

My mother's parents and our brothers came to Great Falls, but I have no memories at all of any of them comforting me. In the faded picture of us taken in front of the morning glories, I stand alone, hands behind my back, trying not to smile. That was the last time I ever saw my grandparents, and it would be another forty years before I met my brothers again.

Margaret took Diane and me to see Mother in a visitation room at Croxford's. The room was named the Sunset room, which I've since come to believe is less offensive than the Slumber Room across the hall. I don't think I looked at Mother's face. I don't remember how she looked, alive or dead. The Sunset Room had chairs covered in ornate tapestry, and Diane asked why there were chairs in the room. Margaret said they were for people to sit in, of course. When we got back to the house, Diane and I were playing around in the laundry room and she asked me how those dead people could sit in the chairs. I thought that was funny; I started laughing and I couldn't stop. Walt slapped me across the face, and said I should be ashamed of myself carrying on like that when my mother had just died.

The family— including me, but not Daddy, because he wasn't family anymore—sat behind the curtain like Billy's family had. I wanted to sit in the church part with my dad, but Margaret wouldn't let me. There were a lot of flowers, and their sweet smell made me feel like I might throw up. The woman behind the curtain sang The Old Rugged Cross. I didn't cry, but I rubbed my eyes a lot so the others would think I was crying or at least that I was trying not to. After the last prayer, the visitors walked past Mother in the casket and looked at her. I watched as Daddy went up, stopped a minute, and then coughed as he hurried out the door. He didn't come to the cemetery. Grandma Johnson and my aunts and uncles, including those from Geraldine, and even Billy s family were there.

We rode in the black hearse to Highland Cemetery, and stood in a circle around the closed casket that would be lowered into the hole after we left. More prayers and lots of tears later, everyone got back into their cars and drove away. I knelt on the back seat of the family funeral car, and looked out the window at the casket until I couldn't see it anymore.

CHAPTER 5—ST. THOMAS

On August 26th 1949, one month and seven days after my eleventh birthday, I became a motherless child. By technical definition I was an orphan, and the events of the next few years supported that theory. Because I was afraid my angry wishes that Mother would die may have materialized, my destiny, in my own troubled mind, became my just desserts. After the funeral, I stayed with Margaret for a week. I tried to stay away from her friends and neighbors who brought casseroles and condolences. Most of them didn't look directly at me, which was fine, but I heard their whispers; "Poor little thing, what will become of her? Her dad's a drunk you know." Or they patted me on the head and told me I would have to be a "big girl now." Mother had hoped she would live long enough for me to grow up. I thought she had. I could even wash my own hair.

After Labor Day, Margaret took Diane to Emerson school for her first day, and she took me to St. Thomas to live. We walked up a long sidewalk to the huge front door of a four-story brick building with the words "St. Thomas Orphanage" written under a cross on the roof.

On the left, past a huge evergreen tree, was a playground but nobody was outside.

We stepped into a vestibule with marble-flooring and a domed ceiling with a skylight. To each side were long empty hallways with ornate dark wooden doors. In front of us, on a twisting staircase with several landings, I saw young children watching us between the spindles.

Margaret pushed a button that summoned a nun who would help with my registration and enrollment.

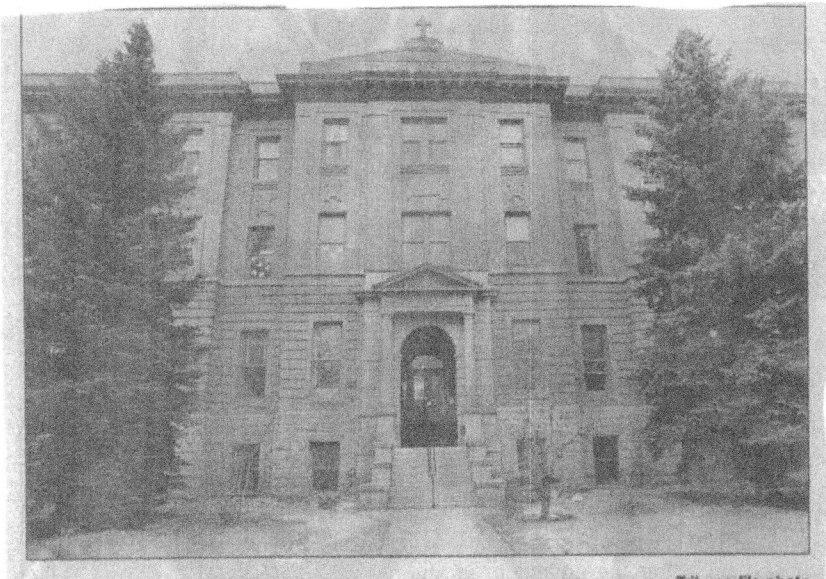

Tribune file photo
The St. Thomas Home opened in 1910, built with donations from a Catholic bishop and the community, on the corner of Central Avenue and 32nd Street North. The building was torn down in 1982.

    The Sisters of Providence wore black habits that made them look like penguins. When Sister Mary Elizabeth introduced herself, she pulled her hands out of the long black sleeves they had been tucked into. The only part of her that was not covered was her face; it was framed with by a roll of white stiff material attached to a skull cap of tight black pleats continuing below her neck. The white covering on her shoulders looked like a cardboard cape. Yards of black material, made up the wide sleeves and the skirts that flowed onto the floor. At her waist, Sister wore a black rosary. That day I gazed in awe of an apparent saint, but later I would laugh at a riddle; "What is black and white and red all over? A wounded Nun."

    Sister gave Margaret some forms to fill out, and Margaret explained that my dad didn't want me to become a Catholic. I didn't know why he said that. Although Mother had been a Catholic, she had never gone to church, and dad had only attended church when he thought he might run for mayor of Great Falls. He made a big public display of my baptism at the Central Christian church on Easter, but after the primary in May, we didn't go back. The one time my dad talked to me about religion was when the two of us were on a fishing trip. One of my cousins in Geraldine was pregnant and another cousin told me she wasn't married. Daddy said he didn't see why the relatives were making such a fuss about her pregnancy. How could they be so sure that her baby wasn't another Christ child? I had attended enough Sunday schools to fear he would be struck by lightening for that comment, and I didn't know how to drive the car.

When I entered the Catholic milieu, I was ripe for conversion. I had had a glimpse of hell when we had left my mother's casket at the cemetery, and I wanted to believe in life after the graveyard. I also was worried about my part in Mother's death. I would come to believe that not only my immediate safety, but perhaps my eternal salvation was dependent on a stamp of approval from the Vatican.

Margaret and I toured the building, from the basement dining room to the fourth floor big girl's dormitory. Big girls were those who were eleven or older, so I would be on the fourth floor. We peeked in the baby room on the first floor, where white metal cribs, each with a high chair at the foot filled the room. Some of the babies were crying, but most were sleeping or quietly staring into the sterile, colorless room. The little girls and boys lived together on the east end of the second floor, which also had some classrooms. The chapel, on the west side of the first floor, could be accessed through the choir balcony from the second floor. In the south part of the basement was a complete laundry room with huge mangles that I would learn to work. The recreation hall, where parties, dances and programs were held, had a curtained stage and a wooden dance floor that the students waxed to a high shine.

The campus, located at the east edge of Great Falls, was quite large. There was a barn, once needed to house the livestock providing food for the orphanage. Large cottonwood trees lined the perimeter of the acreage lending a sense of enclosure.

The big boys, those over eleven, lived in a separate brick building, and they joined the rest of the students for dinner in the main dining room. Their building was separated from the main orphanage by the infirmary.

After we put my belongings in a cupboard that had my name on it, I walked to the end of the sidewalk with Margaret. She hugged me and promised to visit on Saturday. I followed Sister Mary Elizabeth upstairs to the dormitory where she introduced me to Sister John. Although they wore the same outfits, Sister John didn't look like a saint. One night, when I was sick, she came to my bed to give me some medicine without her cap on and I discovered that she had long red hair. Until then, all of us older girls thought the nuns shaved their heads.

Sister John showed me which of the 60 cots, lined up in ten straight rows, would be mine. Margaret had bought me all new underwear and pajamas and the required black shoes. The older girls wore navy-blue jumpers, white blouses, white knee socks, and, if it was cool, a navy blue sweater. Each girl had a navy blue wool tam to wear in church. Before Vatican II, when the Catholic Church made many changes modernizing their practices, all women had to cover their heads when they entered the sanctuary. Sometimes a woman who had forgot her hat would grab a hankie out of her purse to cover her head.

The communal bathroom had sinks on both sides of the long room, and at one end were toilet stalls without doors. Through a doorway was a large shower room with six shower heads. Sister John said I would have to take a shower twice a week, whether I wanted one or not. I would later wish I was required to shower every morning. My bed row used the showers on Monday mornings and Thursday evenings.

Then she took me down to the third floor to the day room. It was like a living room. There were davenports, chairs, desks, and tables with jigsaw puzzles, a large bookcase with board games and books, and an upright piano. All the girls in the room wore the same uniform I had changed into before coming downstairs. Some of them gathered around me asking questions without waiting for my answers.

"What town did you come from? Are you really an orphan or do you have a mother or dad? What grade are you in? Did you bring any candy or gum? You can't have it in the dorm, you know. We have a store. Did you bring money? You better hide it."

The gaggle of navy-blue and white walked me to the dining room at five o'clock. I was assigned a seat at one of the many round tables. I quickly learned that the girls always stood to pray before sitting down, and that they all sat down at the same time, and no one left the dining room until everyone stood to give thanks after the meal.

That evening, we put our tams on and walked two-by-two to the chapel for benediction. I was awestruck by the beauty of the chapel. The altar of white stone had gold-swirl decorated spires reaching to the ceiling. Jesus hung on a cross over the marble altar table that was covered with white linens. A tiny dome-shaped box where the Eucharist was kept was painted in pastel colors with gold trim on the door. Joseph was on one side, and on the other Mary, dressed in a blue and white robe, held baby Jesus. Stained glassed window showed the Stations of the Cross.

Before bedtime, when everyone was in their pajamas, lights were dimmed and the girls knelt beside their cots, facing another statue of Mary, and recited the rosary. Those same rituals were repeated everyday. Others were added during the seasons of advent and lent and The Angeles was said during noon recess.

The first morning I woke up in the room with all those other girls I couldn't remember where I was. I watched and copied what the other girls did. I found my bathroom kit and took a towel from the stack in the corner of the bathroom. I washed my face and brushed my teeth and I dressed in my uniform. After our hair was combed and the beds made, we put our tams on and went to the chapel for daily mass. In those days of the church, members could not receive communion if they had eaten anything, so mass was always before breakfast.

We went to chapel at least twice each day, and I never grew tired of looking at everything there. I learned to dip my fingers in the font of holy water and cross myself before entering the chapel, and to genuflect before sitting in the pew. Some of the girls told me I didn't have to follow the church rules because I wasn't a Catholic, but I wanted to be part of all the ceremonies and rituals. With the help of the book that translated Latin to English, I learned when to stand, sit, or kneel. I loved the smell of incense from a small metal box that hung from a chain that the priest shook around when he first entered the sanctuary. There was a railing that looked like a small fence around the front of the altar, and the Catholics went up to the railing, knelt and put their tongue out to receive the "Body of Christ." I couldn't do that because I wasn't baptized, but I wanted to.

I went to the chapel alone sometimes. I liked the statue of Mary holding the Infant Jesus. If I looked at her real hard I could see her eyes moving. When I lit a candle in one of the colored jars I told myself it was for my mother.

I didn't cry about my mother being gone, but after a few months I wasn't sure if she was really dead. Sometimes I dreamt that she was walking down the gangplank of a large steamer ship. In the dream I would run up to her yelling and she would tell me to stop making a scene. I would shout, "But Mother, I thought you were dead," and she would tell me not to be silly and that I knew she had gone to the old country to visit relatives.

One day during recess, Patsy, the daughter of my mother's friend talked another girl and me into running away. It sounded like a great adventure, and I enjoyed darting behind trees and bushes on our way down Central Avenue. The girls wanted to go to Patsy's mother's apartment first, and then to the other girl's home where her dad lived. They were excited about going home, but as we got closer to town I realized I didn't have anywhere to run to. I walked back to St. Thomas alone. When I walked into my sixth grade class, Sister asked me where I had been. I told her I was going to run away, but I changed my mind. She took me to office of Mother Superior, the boss of everyone in the orphanage except Father. She spanked me and reminded me how lucky I was to have a home, and told me I should ask Jesus to help me be a better person.

Margaret did come back the first Saturday, and lots of times after that. The older kids went home for two days the last weekend of each month, and I went to Margaret's. I looked forward to those visits.

All of the children had chores to do, even the littlest kids. Some of the older girls were assigned to the baby room, a job everyone wanted. The worst job was waxing the dining room floor. We had to put old socks on our hands and smear paste wax on the strips of wood. Then with the rag socks over our shoes we skated around until the wood shone. I had tried ironing my own clothes like some of the other girls did but I just couldn't seem to do it right, so I asked my sister if she would do my laundry. She brought my clothes back each weekend, ironed and folded or on a hanger.

I loved living at St. Thomas until I began wetting my bed. I had never wet my bed before; I didn't know when it happened but I would wake up each morning with soggy sheets. Nothing helped me to stay dry. I tried not drinking any water after supper. I tried wadding my sheet into a ball and stuffing it between my legs; I just peed on that too.

Sister said I was too lazy to get up at night. She would never let me take an extra shower. I tried rinsing my pajamas in the sink each morning and hanging them on my bed to dry, but they still stunk, and my sheets were damp and smelly until Saturday when we got clean bedding. Each day the odor got stronger, and none of the girls came near my bed to visit. No matter how many prayers I said or how many sacrifices— like eating asparagus for the poor souls in purgatory—I made, my bed was still wet each morning. I stopped sucking my thumb when I first came to the school, so the other girls wouldn't know I did that, but after everyone started avoiding my bed, I went back to the comfort of my thumb.

Margaret never mentioned the smelly pajamas I sent home with her each week. She paid my tuition with the stamp machine business that she and Walt took care of, and she made sure I had spending money to buy toothpaste, shampoo, school papers and candy at the school's little store. I had a fun that Halloween and I went trick-or-treating with my niece and nephew. Even though Margaret thought I was getting to big to go, she said I could keep an eye on Diane and Gary, so I collected some candy too. I hid my trick-or-treat goodies under my mattress. I figured no one would try to look under that smelly thing, and I was right.

There were some advantages to being an orphan, especially during the holidays. Do-gooders from town remembered us with parties and gifts. That year I celebrated Christmas as the birthday of Jesus. The chapel was decorated with evergreens and holly, and as the weeks of Advent progressed, the sweet smells of the greens mingled with the smell of hay in the manger. Life sized statues: the Holy Mother, St. Joseph, shepherds, sheep, wise men, camels, and angels circled the empty cradle until midnight-mass when the infant was placed in the crèche.

I spent Christmas with my Lutheran sister and her family. Diane, Gary, and I went to bed on Christmas Eve after leaving cookies for

Santa. We tried to go to sleep so he could sneak through the kitchen door and leave the loot we had asked for. I lay awake on the top bunk listening to my sister and her husband take care of Santa's chores, and I felt warm tears on my face as I wondered where my dad was. I thought of my mother, deep under the frozen Montana prairie, and I wondered about the story of a baby born in a manger to an unwed mother.

I was thrilled to get the real camera I had asked Santa for. I pointed the Brownie at everything that day, including the turkey on the table. Christmas day went by fast, and the next morning I learned that my holiday was over. Margaret helped me pack my bag, and everyone posed so I could finish the film that Margaret promised develop. I was very disappointed, but I didn't let them see me cry. I thanked Margaret when she dropped me off at the orphanage, then I cried. I thought I would be staying with my sister and her family for the holiday school break like most of the other kids who went home for Christmas The only kids left at the orphanage during the holiday were true orphans, who had no family and some of them were invited to homes in town. I called my Grandma Johnson.

She paid for a taxi to come and get me and I stayed with her at the Grand Hotel for the rest of Christmas break. Grandma didn't have a tree, but in the lobby on the first floor of the hotel there was a huge tree with thousands of strands of tinsel on it. It shimmered in the dimly lit room.

Grandma told me that my dad had gone to Alaska after Mother died, and none of the family had heard from him. One of my friends from St. Thomas was visiting her mother who lived at the Grand hotel too, and we had a great time going to movies and window shopping before we had to go back to school.

I began to worry about death— not just about other people dying— but about my own death. One day after lunch I had a head ache and I felt cold and warm at the same time. When the school bell rang I stayed on the couch in the day room; I was drifting in and out of dreams of my mother. The Sisters carried me to the infirmary and the cool sheets of the hospital felt good. I fell back into my dreams, waking up only to take medicine. One night I got out of bed to go the bathroom and I staggered and fell against the wall. The Sisters took me to the hospital in town, and I had an operation to remove my tonsils.

I had been so sure I was dying that I promised Jesus I would become a nun if he would let me grow up. I wanted to be a Catholic in the worst way, but the Sisters kept their promise to my dad that I would not join the church while I was there.

Almost every Saturday evening, I put my tam on and stood in the confessional line with the other girls. Each time, as I slipped into the box with the sliding window that separated the confessor from the priest, I was stopped almost before I could begin.

"Forgive me Father, for I have sinned," I would whisper, and Father would scold, "Carol, you can't be in here." He always sent me to the altar to talk to Jesus about my sins, and I always prayed that I wouldn't die with any sins.

I finally received the sacrament of confession in the spring of 2006. Throughout my life, I attended several protestant churches, including the Universal Church—my favorite because there were ashtrays in the pews—but I yearned for the sacredness that I felt participating in Catholic rituals. I longed for comfort in memorized rituals, rather than outbursts of emotions spurred by the Holy Spirit. There were Vatican barriers, due to marriages in or out of church by my husbands or by me, which kept me from confirmation. After Vatican II, many changes were made. I was finally able to join the church and receive the sacraments, including confession in 1994. However, I went through a class to join the church and along with other initiates participated in a group confession.

Years later, I was early for Mass one Saturday afternoon and discovered that I was in a pew with people waiting to go to confession. I was embarrassed to leave the line, so I braced myself for a private confession. Behind the curtain, after half-expecting to be thrown out, for not wearing something on my head and not being a real Catholic, I finally was able to put a voice to my childish shames. On the way home, I chuckled to myself about finally getting in, and decided to journal about the event. When I opened a page in a journal I pulled out of my desk, I was surprised to find a newspaper clipping I had saved about St. Thomas. I regretted, for only a brief moment, that I had not kept my promise to enter the convent.

When winter seemed over for sure and promises of rebirth were everywhere, I quit wetting my bed. Laura Lee became my best friend.

She didn't have a dad and her mother had to work, so Laura Lee had to stay at St. Thomas. Her breasts almost fit in the bra that belonged to her mother. She let me try it on, but it was too big. We talked about boys and about our changing bodies and I told her what my mother had said about girls bleeding when they became women. We talked about everything: growing up, getting fat, sex, and sins. Laura Lee and I talked a lot about being a bride of Christ.

Summer came, and I rode the orphanage bus to rodeos and the fair. On visits with my sister we went to Ryan Dam for picnics. Sometimes Walt swung Diane, Gary and me through the air until we screamed for him to stop. I stayed with Grandma sometimes and Laura Lee and I went swimming at Mitchell pool or walked down to Broadwater Bay and watched rich people boating on the Missouri. We went to band concerts at Gibson Park and watched families having fun together. The two of us began to see that we were different in ways that made us alike, and we grew even closer. That summer I got a post card with a picture of a Husky dog on it from my dad. It was from Anchorage, Alaska. He wrote that he might be back in the fall.

When I returned to St. Thomas for the seventh grade, the enchantment of being an orphan was gone. I cried most of the time. I begged my grandma to let me live with her. She lived in a small housekeeping room, but she caved into my pitiful pleas. I started junior high at Paris Gibson, a greystone building, named for the founder of Great Falls, that would later become a museum of the arts. Grandma shared her old-age pension with me, and we were classically poor, but poor together. I wondered, in later years, why my sister didn't give Grandma the money from Mother's stamp machines to help pay for my expenses.

Grandma had a great sense of humor, and she loved to tease me. She had sat with me on the steps of the orphanage while I cried and begged her to let me live with her. I had promised to wash her dishes and clean her room every day, if she would just take me home. My promises didn't last long. Grandma bought a figurine of the monkey who could "see no evil." The monkey's hands covered his eyes and grandma painted bright red tears on his cheeks with fingernail polish. The statue sat on the dresser where I had to look at it everyday when I combed my hair, but it didn't bother me. I felt loved in spite of my sins.

CHAPTER 6—ME AND GRANDMA

In 1950, other grandmothers on their way to church—, which Grandma never attended — wore little, pill box hats with veils, gloves, and carried pocketbooks. Now, there are grandmothers, and then there are grandmas. Grandma Johnson was definitely a grandma. She wore black Mary Jane shoes, and although she did wear stockings, she rolled them down and tied a knot just above her knees, which were gnarled like tree burls. Her auburn hair had turned white, and her attempts to dye it resulted in a pink cotton-candy color. She fluffed the wispy tresses around her scalp in an attempt to make her hair seem thicker. When she wore make-up, like on Saturday nights, her lipstick was deep red and she also put some on each cheek and smeared the spot into some "color in her cheeks." Rouge was popular back then. Still is, but today it's called blush.

In the two-and-a-half years that I lived with Grandma, I never knew her to take a bath. She sponge-bathed in the little corner sink in our room and completed her weekend absolutions with a long spray of Evening-in-Paris perfume.

Grandma wore a corset. At one time it had been peach-colored, but was grey from years of use. The contraption, which encased her from her arm pit to below her butt, didn't have a crotch, so Grandma didn't think it needed laundering. Bones, or stays, inserted into the garment like barrel slats held Grandma's flesh firmly together after she fastened one side with multiple hooks-and-eyes. On weekends I watched her go through contortions to tuck herself into the garment. Starting with her thin pendulous breasts, which she rolled up jelly-roll fashion to tuck into the bra, she then squeezed the rest of ample body into the undergarment. She joined the hooks and eyes while pulling any stray fat out of the way. Grandma kept her widow's mite in her cleavage, and never carried a pocketbook.

Grandma's best friend lived a few doors down the hall. She was as tall and thin as Grandma was short and wide. She wore her thick white hair in a bun and when she glided across the floor she reminded me of the Queen of Hearts. She was sophisticated and well read. When she used new words Grandma tried to use the same words. Her friend frequently lost patience with Grandma, like the time they were about to sit down to coffee and Grandma called someone a nonchalant. The Queen of Hearts just got up and glided away before the coffee was even poured. Despite their differences, the friendship lasted many years. Grandma may have wanted to be the lady her friend was, but I think that lady lived vicariously through some of Grandma's antics.

Grandma eked out a living for the two of us on her old age pension and from the iceman's pity. Ice was delivered on Tuesday, and on that day, when I got home from school Grandma gave me money to go to the store to buy pork chops, her favorite food. On other days she sent me, empty handed, to ask the grocer for free pork liver for the cat, or soup bones for our dog. We didn't have any pets. We ate a lot of potato soup that was more soup than potatoes. I was ashamed of my Grandma even before I realized why the iceman left money.

The Grand Hotel was probably one of the finest hotels in Great Falls at the turn of the century. Its opulent past peeked through the faded wallpaper decorated with velvet-looking scrolls. The dark-mahogany banisters recorded years of use with worn paths in the rails. Unoccupied leather divans and club chairs, with tufts of stuffing popping out, showed their age. Our room, on the second floor, was over Woolworth's five and Ten Store on the street level. Four tall, single-paned unscreened windows faced another brick tenement across the alley. Grandma and I slept together in the double bed. We had a table with leaves that folded down, two chairs, a dresser where we kept both dishes and clothes, and a small closet. Grandma's steamer trunk where extras were stored doubled as extra seating. The enamel stove, with chrome trim, had electric burners on one side and the table-level oven was on the other side. The icebox, a wooden cupboard with a tin-lined compartment that held a block of ice was used in the summer only. During the winter we nailed an orange crate to the windowsill outside. We didn't buy ice, but we still had pork chops on Tuesdays. Down the hall were the toilet and a large bathtub that winos slept in sometimes so grandma kept a gallon can under our bed for us to pee in at night. Sometimes she missed the can, and because the floor wasn't level, there would be a puddle in the middle of the room in the morning. Down the hall, around a corner, was a laundry room with a wringer washer and several rinse tubs. Clotheslines, strung across the large room in all directions, drooped with damp laundry until it was the next family's turn to use the laundry. Then the clothes had to be removed even if they weren't dry. We had a radiator that hissed and clanged in the winter as it warmed our room. On bitter cold nights, when ice formed on the inside of our windows, I welcomed the comforting noises of the iron radiator. But I didn't appreciate the brown streaks on my clothes that we tried to dry on it.

Goldie, who used to live near the slough, and her family moved into the hotel and the boys and I became a trio of redheads that menaced downtown Great Falls. Central Avenue and the alleys were our playgrounds. There were four movie theaters in town and every time they changed the marquee we were in line for the nine-cent matinee. It was cheap babysitting for families trying to get along in one or two rooms.

The boys and I made slingshots and used bobby pins to pop balloons in Woolworth's and Newberry's. When the department store across the street put in the city's first escalator, we were there to ride it up and down, over and over, until we were asked to leave. We collected huge refrigerator crates and built clubhouses in the alley. We forced the gravity-balanced fire escapes above the alley to come down by walking out to the ends. There we tried smoking and shared what we knew about sex.

The first time I smoked I got so sick that I went back to my room, crawled into bed and promised God if he would just let me live I would never smoke again. But with practice, I got better at it and I didn't keep my promise until 1982.

The boys sold newspapers, and they showed me how to get started. I had my corner on Central Avenue. The afternoon paper was called the

Leader. We bought a bundle of the orange afternoon paper at the back door of the Tribune building, and sold them at a fixed rate for a small profit. I held the front page of the paper high in the air, shouting the headlines to entice people to read the rest of the story. I usually sold all my papers before the boys.

Starting junior high was scary for me. While most of the kids were coming from grade schools with more than one sixth grade, I had been in a classroom of only eleven kids. Paris Gibson Junior High had hundreds of kids. My cousin was starting seventh grade too, but we didn't have the same home rooms. Some of the boys in my class were from prominent Great Falls families. I thought of them as rich kids. Dennis Croxford's dad owned the mortuary. The Guan boys, whose family was rumored to be with the Mafia, owned the Park Hotel. Another boy was the son of a jeweler with a store on Central. In a few weeks I adjusted to changing classes and fighting for a place in the crowded halls. I made new friends, one of whom was a midget, just like the Munchkins in the Wizard of Oz. She was only about three feet tall. She seemed happy all the time, and she was very popular, so I was too when I was with her. One of the bigger boys packed her from class-to-class on his shoulder, the rest of us followed along like a queen's court of jesters.

Our home room had a meeting every Friday called home-room club. We learned Robert's Rules of Order and practiced conducting meetings, but we also took turns providing the entertainment of the day. When my turn to entertain came around I sang a cowboy song and the rowdy boys in the back of the room clapped and whistled. It wasn't long before they asked me to do the entertainment again. The next time I wore my fringed cowgirl skirt and western boots. I sang "The Strawberry Roan." They were making fun of me. At first, I was angry with the boys; later I was ashamed of myself for letting them use me for their amusement.

One of the girls in my class had a cat. When the cat had kittens she talked me into taking one of the babies home. I was happily surprised when Grandma agreed I could keep the coal-black ball of fur. I named him Smoky, after a horse in one of my favorite movies. The kitten became my constant companion; Grandma seemed to enjoy him too. Smokey tolerated a collar, but fought a leash. He sat on my shoulder when I ran around town and accepted an occasional pat from people who were drawn to the girl with the black cat. At night Smokey slept on my side of our bed, and sucked on the corner of my pajama collar. When I ran on the linoleum in the hallway and turned abruptly into our room he slid on his claws past the door and scrambled to follow me inside.

Daddy came back to Montana before Christmas. He slept on the floor in our room until got his own place. My dad teased me about my cat and said it was time for me to be thinking about getting a real boy friend, but I knew he was just kidding. Besides, most of the boys I knew were nasty and rude. Corky, one of the boys who lived at the Grand, purposely bumped into my chest. When I winced with pain he said, "they" were supposed to hurt because "they" were beginning to grow. Sometimes, while I was taking a bath, I sucked my tummy in as far as I could, but my ribs still were higher than the knobs on my chest.

My passage from little girl to teenager was not smooth. One day I was putting doll clothes on Smoky, and the next day I was stealing my dad's cigarettes. One day I was shaving the fuzz on my legs, dragging Daddy's razor through the lather I worked up with the brush in his shaving mug, and the next day I was sitting on a saddle in the basement of Monkey Wards pretending I was a cowgirl.

Christmas came to downtown Great Falls in early November, when the city hung garlands across Central Avenue and department stores put lighted trees on their mezzanines. I thought the song "Silver Bells" had been written for Great Falls. The people from the Salvation Army, dressed in their navy-blue uniforms, played Christmas music on the corners and they rang bells to remind people to drop extra coins in their pots for the poor. Santa Claus came to the Civic Center party and gave out sacks of candy and oranges to everyone there.

With money Daddy gave me, I bought a real tree that we sat on our trunk. We decorated it with a string of bubble lights and lots of tinsel; we all agreed it was beautiful. I even hung some socks on the side of the trunk for Santa to fill. Uncle Teddy, a strange kind of Santa, came from the winter sheep camp. He was, as usual, generous with his money for as long as it lasted. He bought a hat and scarf set for me, and my sock was filled with nuts, candy canes and an orange. Grandma made divinity candy and baked a chicken he bought and Aunt Goldie brought pies when her family came across the hall.

We had an old-fashioned family holiday until Uncle Teddy drank too much of Daddy's whiskey. He was what people called a mean drunk. Uncle Teddy got it into his head that Smokey had eaten a piece of the chicken on his plate, and he tried to grab the cat. When the cat dashed under our bed, Uncle Teddy turned on me. He pulled off his belt with a big metal buckle. While Daddy and Uncle Toppy were trying to grab him, Grandma screamed at me to run and hide. I stayed in the laundry room until I heard the men walk down the stairs, and the big door of the hotel slam behind them.

I hated it when my family drank whiskey or beer. Their drinking ruined everything that was fun. Grandma drank too. She dressed up on weekends and went to the Lobby Bar down the street from our hotel. My cousins and I went into the bar and we found her sitting at a table with a bunch of Air Force boys. They bought her drinks and she danced with them. It looked like they were all having fun, but I felt the same kind of shame for her that I had felt for myself when the boys in the home room class made fun of me.

That winter Uncle Teddy broke his leg at the sheep camp and had to stay with Daddy. He hated the plaster cast and soaked it off twice. My dad was always mad at Uncle Teddy, his youngest brother, for one thing or another. One of Daddy's stories about Uncle Teddy's involved a pot of white beans that Daddy was cooking in their room. He had left the beans simmering on the stove while he went somewhere, and when he came back he caught Teddy sweeping up the beans that had boiled over onto the floor into a dust pan, and pouring them back into the pot on the stove. Uncle Teddy and Daddy just couldn't seem to get along. Grandma wanted Uncle Teddy to sleep on our floor, but I was afraid he would kill my cat or me. The second time he soaked the cast off his broken leg he didn't even go back to the doctor. Grandma was sure her baby would be crippled for life, but Uncle Teddy's life ended before his bone healed. In one of his drunken stupors he crawled onto the concrete railing on the third level of a parking garage. He rolled off and crushed his skull on the concrete below. Grandma mourned for her boy who never grew up, never became a man, and in her mind, never had a chance in life. She choked on bitter tears as we rode in the hearse from Croxford's to Highland cemetery. When we left Teddy's casket sitting by the mound of dirt, Daddy held Grandma up as she staggered back to the car.

For awhile after Teddy's funeral, Daddy drank more than usual. One time I was with him at the Glenwood when he kept playing the same song on the juke box and I saw tears running through the lines in his leathery face. He said he missed my mother all the time. I never thought much about Mother that year, and I still had no tears.

When the snow melted and the roads to Geraldine opened up, Daddy and I visited his friends who owned Rusty's bar. Their ranch looked like the setting for some of my favorite western movies. We drove to the base of the Highwood Mountains west of Geraldine As we climbed higher wheat fields gave way to rolling hills with groves of still bare Aspens gathered in the ravines. The ranch, in a box-canyon, was surrounded by snow capped rocky peaks. The sprawling one-story split-log structure had the expected stone chimney, and several yards behind the house stood a picture-perfect barn and corral.

The ranchers raised palomino horses. One of their thoroughbreds mated with an unregistered quarter horse and they gave me the bastard colt. Trigger, which of course I named him, had the color and markings of the palomino mare. He was still a little unsteady on his gangly legs when we arrived and his velvet-soft muzzle poked my face when I bent down to hug him. I had no place to keep the horse, but he was mine, and with that gift came the invitation to come back any time we could.

In June, one of Montana's notorious late snow storms passed through Montana; my colt ran blindly into a barbed wire fence. They had to put him down. We didn't return to the ranch that summer or ever again. The entire family was killed years later when they were in an accident with their private plane.

Two of Daddy's brothers who lived in Oregon came to Montana for Teddy's funeral and uncle Tuffy, who never married, suggested that Daddy bring their mother to Oregon to live. With the promise of new beginnings, Grandma and I eagerly packed everything we owned into her steamer trunk. I snuck Smokey onto the Empire Builder in a cardboard hat box, and tried to shush his mewing when the train began creaking and rocking across the trestle carrying us across the Missouri River. Twenty-four hours later when we crossed the Willamette River in Oregon, the conductor threw the urine-soaked box out of the train, and told me to hide the cat until we got off. Grandma and I took a taxi to the Greyhound depot and when we got on the bus we made our way back to the very last seat.

Portland, Oregon, the biggest city I had ever seen, was nestled within forested hills. There were tall buildings that shot up into the sky farther than I could see from my seat on the bus. When we got off the bus in Canby, I pulled my kitty out from under my shirt and said to the driver, "Bet you didn't know I had this." I was so excited about arriving that his reply, "Bet you wouldn't have ridden my bus if I had known," didn't dampen my high spirits.

Daddy and Uncle Tuffy rented a house that was in the middle of a grove of fruit trees with cherries waiting to be picked and the promise of pears, apples and peaches in the fall. Grandma and I had never bought fruit when we lived in Montana, except at Christmas time. A small, fenced pasture was behind the house and a barn for a cow. Or maybe a horse? The living room was bigger than our one-room home at the Grand Hotel. The bathroom was off a small bedroom on the main floor that Daddy and Uncle Teddy would share. Upstairs was another small bedroom and an unfinished attic. We had a dining room and a large kitchen that had a porch where we found a wringer washer. No matter that we would have to hang our laundry outside in the constant winter rain; no matter that the rain rinsed items would have to be draped in front of the oil stove in the dining room; we had our very own washing machine. No matter that Grandma and I had to walk through the men's bedroom to get to the bathroom; there were no winos sleeping in our tub anymore. Grandma kept her pee can under her bed that she sat up on some plywood in the unfinished attic so I could have a room of my very own. We were rich!

Uncle Tuffy worked at a shingle mill, and he gave Grandma money for groceries. Daddy helped her too, when he won.

Uncle Tuffy was short and stocky; his arms bulged with muscles from years of hard work. His arms seemed to be attached wrong because his elbows pointed outward and they never really hung straight down. His legs were bowed like his arms. After Teddy died, he was Grandma's youngest, so she took to babying him as much as he would let her. I liked Uncle Tuffy, but there was something about him that scared me.

The four Johnson children who lived in Oregon included Joe, Rose, Edith, Tuffy and their families. Uncle Joe and Aunt Helen had two kids, Joann and Kenny. They were probably the most normal family in Grandma's brood. Helen was a housewife and Joe worked at the lumber mill. They spent a lot of time with their children and kept to themselves. When Joann and I graduated from the eighth grade, Uncle Tuffy bought us identical wrist watches. Joann had to keep hers on her mother's dresser except for dress up occasions. I got to wear mine all the time, and I lost it before the summer was over.

Edith, Grandma's youngest daughter, had been in a tuberculosis sanitarium for a couple of years and had just returned home. She had to stay in bed all the time except to go to the bathroom, her husband, who also worked, did all the cooking. Her boys, who were younger than I was, did the laundry and housecleaning. I liked to go to their house and help with the housework because Aunt Edith had a parakeet that she had taught to do tricks and talk. What I remember most about Aunt Edith is that she looked like her parakeet. Her mouth was small and tight and the Johnson nose, which didn't look bad on my uncles, was thin and sharp in the middle of her drawn face.

Grandma's other daughter, Rose, lived in Portland—I never met her—and I heard she had married one of Grandma's boyfriends.

I loved living in Oregon. I picked crops with Joann and Kenny like almost all kids in Oregon did so they could buy their own school clothes. We climbed onto the farmer's bus before the sun came up and worked in the fields until about two each afternoon. It was hard, dirty, and hot work but I had money of my very own. Grandma took me on the bus—without the cat—to Oregon City, and I had more clothes than I had since Mother died.

The Canby school went from first through eighth grade. I made new friends, and quickly became one of the leaders of our little group. I discovered that having an A posted on the bulletin board for everyone to see felt good, and I worked hard for that spotlight among my peers. We were learning about unions and strikes in the social studies class; I led the girls in our class on a strike for the right to wear slacks to school. We made posters and marched around the school grounds until a local newspaper brought too much publicity to the situation and the teachers agreed to negotiate. After that, girls could wear slacks to school every Friday.

Another time, several of my friends and I had skipped class to practice a musical production we were creating. We were in the girls' bathroom when the principal walked in. We figured we were in big trouble, but he encouraged us to continue with the play without skipping class, and he let us practice on the gymnasium stage. We stayed after school and practiced during lunch time. When we performed our little musical for the entire student body I got special recognition for screenwriting and directing.

Christmas in Oregon was crepe paper draped from corner to corner of our living room, a real tree that touched the ceiling, caroling with cousins, neighbors playing their fiddles and Grandma's divinity and fudge.

One of the ways that Daddy supplemented the household income was to host a poker game in our dining room every Wednesday. On those nights Grandma served coffee and homemade cookies before climbing the stairs to her plywood area in the attic. The longer the games lasted and the drunker the men got, the harder it was for Grandma and me to sleep. One Wednesday, after Grandma had hollered down the stairs and asked them to quiet down several times, she lost her temper. She jumped out of her bed and stomped on the floor above the poker table. Her foot went through the ceiling right above the table. While Daddy helped free her, the others cashed in their chips and the game was over early that night.

Another spring and another promise of a horse of my own. Daddy and I drove to a nearby town to look at a horse for sale. The seller of the older bay agreed to hold the horse until Friday. Daddy gave her $25 and told her we would return at the end of the week. The plan was that Daddy would drive me out to get the horse which I would ride the fifteen miles back to Canby. The poker game on Wednesday didn't go well for my dad, and we never went to get the horse.

Things seemed to go from bad to worse from then on. Uncle Tuffy had complained several times about Smokey being in the house. I had trained the cat to scratch on my dormer window at night so I could let him in to sleep with me. Uncle Tuffy discovered that I had been letting the cat in and he brooded about it until one day, in a drunken rage, he shot my cat. I hadn't seen Smokey for a couple of nights and searched everywhere for him, calling him and asking everyone if they had seen him. No one told me what happened until I found Smokey in the dirt under the house. I could barely hear him crying, but I followed the noise through the spider-webbed darkness with a flashlight. He didn't lift his head when I talked to him and then I saw the dried blood. I put him on my jacket and dragged him into an open area. I offered him a milk-soaked rag to suck on, but he just lay there breathing hard. I cried and prayed but when I came home from school the next day, Smokey was gone. Grandma said they had put him out of his misery.

When I started crying, I couldn't stop. I didn't feel like eating, and I slept fitfully each night after I cried myself to sleep. I wanted my cat and I wanted my mother! My grades plummeted, I lost weight, and I hated Oregon and everything about it, especially the constant rain that cried with me.

Then one day the principal called me to his office. He told me there had been a problem at home, and that I was to get off the school bus at my neighbor's house. It was a long ride home that day. I couldn't imagine what could be so wrong that I couldn't even go home. When I saw broken furniture in my yard, I thought there had been a fire. I was scared about Grandma until I saw her coming across the road. She said Daddy and Uncle Tuffy had gotten into a fight over the rent payment and broke some things. I could some of the windows were broken too. Grandma hugged me and told me everything would be all right. I helped her nail some cardboard over the windows, and we threw the broken furniture in the barn. There were pieces of broken dishes all over the house, and Tuffy had even torn the phone off the wall. My dad was unable to tear the toilet off the floor, but he had tried and the seat to the toilet was in the bathtub.

Not long after that, Daddy and Uncle Tuffy were arguing again and Tuffy slammed out of the house at night, heading for the tavern down the road. When we heard brakes squealing, Daddy said, "Well, he just about had time to reach the highway." My dad lived to regret that sarcasm because Tuffy was hit by a car that night and died a couple of days later. Grandma had to bury another son and it wasn't any easier on her the second time. Grandma and I both wanted to go home.

My period started on my graduation day, and although I had been told it would happen someday I didn't believe it until I saw the blood on my panties. Grandma gave me some money, and told me to stop and buy some Kotex and a sanitary belt before I went to graduation practice. I went to the practice first thinking no one would know because I was wearing jeans. That night, as I dressed for the ceremony, when I put on my first pair of nylons, held up with my first garter belt beneath the sanitary belt that held the Kotex, I knew I wasn't going to like being a woman very much.

As my classmates and I gathered behind the stage curtain, I noticed a brown streak on my chair. Just as I switched chairs, the boy who was to be my partner in the Pomp and Circumstance march walked up. I explained that there was something on the chair and he said—in a way that told me he knew what it was—"I saw it."

Grandma and I boarded the train in Portland and looked forward to crossing the continental divide that separated us from our heartland.

CHAPTER 7—CONTINENTAL DIVIDES

Grandma and I ate breakfast in the dining car, enjoying the silver creamers and linen napkins more than the oatmeal, which was the cheapest thing on the menu. The train snaked around curves above the glacier-green river below, and passed through dry snow sheds. At Marias Pass the creaking of the climb gave way to a rocking descent as we crossed the continental divide and dropped down to rolling grasslands.

The southbound route paralleled the Rocky Mountain Front. Purple mountains' majesty sang in my mind as I thrilled at seeing the totems of my homeland. At the outskirts of Great Falls we passed slowly through freight yards, and I spied the slough my cousins had lived near. The train slowed to a stop at the Great Northern station next to the Civic Center. When we stepped off the train, I looked straight down First Avenue south—skid row—and I brushed away tears of happiness as I embraced the familiarity of childhood landmarks.

Grandma called a couple of her friends, and by evening we had a home. Another housekeeping room with the bathroom down the hall, but it felt like home. We were upstairs in an old brownstone house that had once been a single-family home. Grandma's friend, Stella, lived in three rooms on the main floor and an older couple had a two-roomer upstairs. We slept on the floor the first night because Grandma sprayed the mattress for bedbugs, which was necessary, but we had to share the room with cockroaches. We heard them scratching across the floor as they scurried out of sight whenever we turned on a light. We learned to be careful with sugar and other crumbs; Grandma made the room homey with curtains and a begonia in the window.

Margaret and Walt had moved from public housing into a brand new house east of town. Diane and Gary were school age and Margaret worked part-time at Woolworth's. Mother had left a trust fund for me, and there was another seven hundred dollars set in reserve for when I turned 18. Margaret helped me through the legal maze so that I could draw out some of the seven hundred for high school expenses An appointed trustee approved requests to draw money from the account. According to my dad, there had been close to five thousand dollars in an account earmarked for my college education. Dad said there was no way Walt, a carpenter who was laid off each winter, made enough money to buy a brand new house. My sister agreed that Mother had left a lot more than seven hundred for me, but she claimed my dad and some crooked attorney drained the fund. I was just glad there was, what I thought of as a lot of money, left.

I learned to appreciate just how much one hundred dollars was when Daddy and I went to Geraldine to work during the harvest. Daddy taught me to drive the old farm trucks. My cousin Larry—who I never liked much because he always talked nasty and wanted to play sex games—drove one truck, and I drove the other. We hauled wheat from the combine, where our uncles were threshing in the fields, to the grain elevator in town. Larry hadn't changed a bit and he kept begging me to let him be my first boyfriend. Every time he started in I told him I had my period. I hated my period, the Kotex, and the sanitary belts. I dreaded it coming because working in the fields was so hot and itchy anyway. When I didn't have a period in August I bragged to my dad that I had wished it away. He yelled at me and slapped me across the face. I went to Aunt Eula who told my dad that my periods would be irregular for awhile. Daddy apologized, but things were different between us after that. Dad slapped me again the first time I wore some lipstick. When we left Geraldine, Daddy told me he would hold onto the money Uncle Hobart had paid me so it wouldn't get lost, but he got rolled by some chippie; or so he said, and I never got any of that money.

All of a sudden everything about my family seemed wrong; I was ashamed of them. I cursed at Grandma for wiping her nose on the hem of her dress, or drinking out of our water pitcher.

Aunt Goldie got pregnant; Uncle Toppy got a divorce. Goldie took my cousins to live in Lewistown before her baby was born. She told Grandma she didn't care what color the baby turned out to be; she was keeping it.

That year, my friend, Laura Lee introduced me to a girl named Barbara. We were all fourteen years old and ready to be teenagers. We went roller skating almost every day. The attraction at the roller rink was boys, actually soldiers. The young airmen from the East Base, many of them teenagers themselves, were not at the roller rink to skate. I met a boy named Danny who walked me home one night. When I stopped in front of the row of brownstones and pointed to the room where I lived he thought I was kidding, but then he got real serious and told me to stay away from the roller rink because I was a nice kid, and I was going to get into big trouble. I kept going to the roller rink, but I never saw him again. Once when I was skating with a boy, I saw my dad dodging his way across the rink. He grabbed me by my long hair, pulled me across the floor and out of the building. I just wanted to die. I cried all the way home. I hated him for shaming me like that.

Barbara and I became best friends. She was poor too, but she lived in a house. She was the oldest of seven brothers and sisters. Although their home was crowded and there were ten plates at the dinner table to fill, Barbara's mother always made me feel welcome.

Great Falls High, with its brick collegiate-style building, seemed daunting to me. Barbara and I didn't have poodle skirts and saddle oxfords like most of the girls who wore different colored angora sweaters with matching sox each day. Some of the older kids even had their own cars. Boys with ducktail haircuts and football letter jackets whistled at us; at first we didn't realize they were making fun of us.

I tried to keep up my grades, but Barbara and I knew we didn't fit into the high school crowd. We dated guys from the Base whom the hometown boys hated. Barbara was a beautiful native American with high cheekbones and thick black hair. While I was still freckled, my red hair had turned a pretty auburn and the Johnson nose made me look older. We had no trouble finding dates. On weekends, we walked up and down Central Avenue, stopping at cafes to drink cherry cokes and eat free soda crackers. I met a flyboy named Whitey. He was older, and had an old hearse for a car. There were curtains on the long windows of the car, which could hold a lot of kids and a lot of beer. Holter Dam, thirty miles out of Great Falls, seemed a safe distance from police and parents for us to hold our keggers. We danced on the concrete slabs left from the dam's construction, with music blasting from the car radios. When we got back to town we stayed at each others' houses to sleep off the booze.

Grandma tried to put a stop to my weekend adventures. She suspected we were not popping corn and drinking hot cocoa anymore, and one time when she found out where the party was going to be she called the police. They came and took Barbara and me, the only ones underage, home in the squad car. Barbara's mother told the police that her daughter had her permission to be at that party, and as long as she wasn't drinking it was none of their business. She told the police to take Barbara back to the party, and they did! Grandma was sitting on the bed when I walked into our room between two officers. I screamed at her for calling the police on me. I was expecting a ride back to the party like Barbara, but the officer tightened his grip on my arm and told me to shut up. He said he never heard a child talk to an adult that way, and he didn't want to hear another word out of me or I would go to juvenile hall. I shut up and sat down by Grandma, and listened to his lecture about respecting my elders and helping my grandmother instead of causing her trouble. After the police left, I lit into Grandma big time. I told her I was going back to that party, and she better not call the police again if she knew what was good for her. I went back and she didn't call the police.

Although Christmas was very sad. I was in love with the.twenty-three-year- fly-boy with the platinum-colored hair. Daddy didn't come around and Grandma didn't do anything to celebrate; we had no tree, no gifts, and nothing special for dinner. On Christmas Eve, Whitey, Barbara and her boyfriend and I, went to another girl's house and for a party while her parents were out for the evening. They had a beautiful tree, and we sat around with just the tree lights on, necking and listening to Christmas music on the radio. Whitey and I walked back to my place as large, soft snowflakes began to fall. It seemed like such a beautiful night. We sat on the inside steps and did some heavy petting for the first time. Grandma leaned over the railing several times to tell me to come to bed; the last time she told me to get my ass upstairs or else. It was daylight on Christmas morning 1952 when Whitey asked me to marry him.

My January report card was all red Fs and I didn't care. Whitey wanted to marry me, he called me Ma, and I called him Pa. Of course, once Whitey and I crossed the line with heavy petting it was only a matter of time until we went all the way. At least I thought we had.

Daddy was angry about my failing grades and especially about any plans to get married, especially to a service boy. We had terrible fights. One evening he held me against the wall, and every time I refused to go back to school, he slammed me into the wall. Before he broke down and gave me permission to marry Whitey, he hit me with a cast iron skillet. Then Grandma made him quit fighting with me.

I Margaret to help me with my wedding. At first she argued and pleaded with me to wait at least a year but eventually she decided that if I was married I would have a home, and it might be better than living with my grandmother who had no control over me. We went to the courthouse to see the district judge. I needed his signature to remove all the money from my trust fund. We met with him in his private chambers. He asked why I needed that much money. I told him I was going to get married and wanted to buy a dress, and some other things for my wedding. The judge smiled and looked at me incredulously.

"How old are you?"

"Fourteen"

He looked at Margaret and asked her if she realized I was too young for a marriage license. She started to answer him, but I butted in and assured him that my dad had given me permission. He lowered his bushy eyebrows over his eyes and glared at me.

"I can give my five year old daughter permission to get married, but in Montana you have to be at least sixteen. Have you had sexual relations with your boyfriend?"

I hesitated answering, but then I thought if I said yes he would have to let me get married.

"And how old did you say your boyfriend is?"

"Twenty-three, and he has a good job in the Air Force," I reassured the judge.

"Good God!" he roared at my sister, "What were you thinking bringing this child here for permission to get married?"

Margaret tried to explain that I was pretty much on my own, and that my dad was not supervising me and Grandma was unable to control me. I was running wild, and she thought it would be better if I settled down early.

I told the judge that I was in love with Whitey, and I would just run away and marry him anyway if he didn't say I could.

He pushed an intercom button, and when a woman answered, the judge asked her to come to his office. Almost before I could understand what was happening, the matron handcuffed me. She led me out of the building and into the back of a government car. She took me to the juvenile detention center where I stayed for the next fourteen days. I was examined, interrogated, and not allowed to have any visits from Whitey.

The woman who worked at the center encouraged me to spend time in the kitchen with her. She offered to help me make cookies, but I couldn't stop crying. The room I slept in wasn't locked, but the front door was. There were other cots in the room, but I was the only girl there at that time. My dad never came to see me; Grandma called and told me she was talking to some people to see if I could live with them; Marge brought me new pajamas and magazines. At the county health department, a lady doctor talked to me before she made me spread my legs; then she felt inside me. I went to the courthouse and talked with two men for a long time. They asked questions about what Whitey and I had done. I didn't know about most of the things they asked.

"Did you wrap your legs around him? Was he on the top or bottom? Did you sit on him? Did it hurt when he went in you? Describe where your legs were. How long did you have intercourse? How many times?"

I wanted to die right there in that room.

The doctor said there was no penetration. I wasn't pregnant. I was disappointed. Whitey and I had talked about having lots of kids, and I had hoped that if I was pregnant the judge would change his mind.

During the second week I was locked up my sister and I met again with the judge. She told him that my father had a drinking problem and his behavior with me was probably inappropriate. She said my dad had tried to rape her when she was my age, and that she had to go to live with her real father. I screamed at her that she was wrong about my dad, and that I didn't believe her. She said horrible things about Grandma, and she said her husband didn't want me living with them. She said maybe it would be best if I went to the girls' reform school. I couldn't believe she said that! My dad and my grandma had asked a couple of mother's friends if they could take me. The judge told Margaret that based on the interviews and medical examinations I had lied about being sexually active. He said that the young man I had accused could have been dishonorably discharged from the Air Force and even sent to jail. He said it appeared that I was incorrigible and that it would be difficult for a new family to bond with me. He agreed with my sister that I should be placed in the Montana State Girls' reform school.

I ran out of tears before Marge brought me a suitcase and some new clothes. She told me to try to take advantage of the opportunities at the school, and to write to her. It would be a long, long time before I cried again.

I was married and had five children before I heard from Whitey again. He had called Aunt Goldie to get my phone number. He told me he still wanted to marry me, and that he had a good job setting pins in a bowling alley in Wisconsin. He was thirty-two at that time. What a golden opportunity I missed.

CHAPTER 8—HELENA VALLEY

The Montana State Vocational School for girls, better known as the girls' reform school, was located on the northern flats of Helena, Montana's capitol city. That February of 1953 I rode, through the Missouri river canyon where my dad and I had fished so many times, in a state car with two strangers who had come to the detention hall to pick me up after breakfast on Monday morning. The driver didn't speak at all as he put my box of belongings in the trunk, but an older lady said I could call her Mrs. Burns. She opened the back door of the car and told me to get in. After she locked the door, she said the trip to Helena would take about two-and-a-half hours; we would stop at Wolf Creek to use the bathroom. I might just have well been locked in a rocket to the moon. Everything and everyone I'd ever known was being left behind, and I was traveling into an unknown future. I imagined the worse as I wondered what the reform school would be like and how I would be treated. I thought of jumping out of the car and running when we stopped, but to where? Everyone had decided where I should be, and how I should be. I felt futureless. Whitey, who had said he loved me and wanted to marry me, disappeared after I was arrested. Did my dad really try to rape Margaret? Was that why she went away when I was a baby? Is that why she was always asking me if my dad touched me funny? How come my dad didn't come to see me in the detention center? Why did Mother really die? Poor Grandma, at least she had tried to give me a home, and I messed that up. The woman talked to me a little about the scenery and other things, but after a few of my one-word replies she quit trying.

Helena, Montana, sits deep in a valley. Interstate 5 crested over mountains and then dropped down into miles of straight-as-an-arrow highway that ended near the copper-domed state Capitol but we turned off before reaching the city.

Helena Valley High School, the name entered on graduation certificates of those girls matriculating out of the reform school, was surprisingly beautiful. Several red-brick cottages sat among cottonwood trees and a frozen creek bed, banked with last fall's cattails and willows, lazed across the campus. As we approached the administration building, bluish-green winter mountains were visible in the background.

A tall grey-haired lady came out to meet us. Miss Miller, the superintendent of the school, greeted me with a firm handshake. She thanked the women for bringing me safely to the school. I picked up my box and followed Miss Miller into the building. She spoke softly, and looked directly at me. Miss Miller invited me to sit down in a chair next to another woman whom she introduced as Miss Virginia, the dean of the school. Miss Miller's hair was secured in a roll on the back of her head and she wore wire-rim glasses low on her nose so she could use them when she was writing, but she looked over them when she was talking to me. She had tiny rivulets above her mouth into which some of her lipstick had leaked. Miss Virginia, who I would learn was called Miss Vagina by the inmates, was large, not fat, just big. She wore brown oxfords with black anklets that showed under her tweed slacks. She cut her hair like a man.

They asked me questions about Whitey, my grandma, my dad, and my grades. Miss Miller showed me around the building, and explained that although her office and living quarters on the first floor were off limits to students, the rest of the building was classrooms. She said I would continue in the ninth grade for the rest of the year.

"How long will I have to stay here?" I asked.

"That will depend on how well you get along, your grades and what plans you have for the future. Some girls stay until they graduate, but most girls stay about one year."

Miss Virginia asked, "Where would you go anyway?"

"I guess back to my grandma's."

"Well, that didn't work out too well for you or your grandmother, now did it?" she asked, but it wasn't really a question.

Miss Miller showed me the auditorium upstairs where there were band instruments. She said if I was interested in taking music lessons I could earn that privilege. Before Miss Virginia escorted me to my assigned cottage, Miss Miller asked, "Do you smoke, Carol?"

"Oh, no," I lied.

The cottage had windows with fancy wrought-iron bars that didn't look like bars. Several girls scattered from the windows when Miss Virginia put her key into the locked front door. I was handed over to the house matron, Miss Susan, and Miss Virginia went down the hall to her private quarters on the west side of the building. Miss Susan was young and pretty. She was wearing slacks and a sweater. She led me upstairs to a hall that had many open doorways. Each opened into a tiny bedroom. I left my box of things in a room and Miss Susan showed me around and introduced me to some of the girls. On the main floor, there was a small piano room and a large day room, furnished with couches of various sizes and overstuffed chairs. Some girls were doing jigsaw puzzles. French doors opened into a dining room with checker-clothed tables. A dishwashing pantry was separated from the food preparation area by a swinging door. Miss Susan told me all girls were assigned to chores and the assignments rotated the first of each month. She said I would start in the pantry after breakfast the next day.

The basement had several automatic washing machines that could be used anytime and there were the six showers. Miss Susan said the showers were very busy each morning, so I might want to try bathing in the evenings at first. She gave me some state underwear and pajamas and two dresses to wear until my clothes were marked.

"Then you can keep your clothes and wear what ever you like as long as it is appropriate, or you can wear the state dresses. A lot of the girls do wear the dresses. The rules about smoking are simple. You can only smoke in the day room at the time the cigarettes are passed out. If you are caught smoking anywhere else on the campus, or at any other time, your smoking privileges will be taken away from you. We will give you half of a king size cigarette after each meal, and after school, and again in the evening before bedtime, which is nine on school nights and ten on weekends."

"O great", I thought to myself and wondered how I could get on the smoking list.

"Well, actually," I quietly offered, "I do smoke, but I was afraid to admit it when Miss Miller asked me."

"You're not the first girl to lie about that," laughed Miss Susan. As long as you have money to pay for the cigarettes you can be on the approved list. She told me she would clear it up with Miss Miller and I made a mental note to make sure Margaret sent me enough allowance each month to cover my "needs."

In 2002, when the State of Montana received the tobacco settlement monies, I challenged Montana, with no success, to give some of that money to kids like me who became addicted at an early age with the help of the State.

The girls I sat with for supper seemed just like girls from any of the schools I had been to. Some introduced themselves and asked questions and others kept their eyes on their plates of food. Many of the girls in the dining room had shiny black hair either braided or worn very long. The darker skin and high cheekbones identified them as Indian girls, who came from the many reservations around the state. One of my dinner partners was an Indian girl named Regina. She was very nice about telling me what to expect for the rest of the evening; she advised me to stay away from a couple of girls that were known to be tough, and which matrons were the strictest. I didn't have to wash dishes that evening so while I waited for the cigarette pass, I went up to my room and put some of my things away. I noticed some of the girls had decorated their rooms with posters and family pictures. Some even had fancy bedspreads on their cots and throw rugs on the floor. I just hoped I wouldn't be there that long. When I went to bed that night I looked out through the mesh wire in my window at a cracked moon and prayed I would wake up from a bad dream.

Although my arrival at the girl's school was not a dream, it wasn't really a nightmare either. The girls at the school were between the ages of nine and eighteen and their crimes ran the gamut of homicide to incorrigibility. Half of the girls at the school were from reservations in Montana. Whenever an Indian girl was admitted we almost always had to be deloused with kerosene shampoo. I got along with most of the girls and learned if I held the half a cigarette we were given with a bobby pin I could smoke it down to the very last part.

I secured my place in the pecking order of the cottage I lived in during the first week when one of the girls tried to pick a fight with me. I didn't want to fight and I was as surprised when I jumped up and ran after the bully. She ran into the pantry and I grabbed her by the back of her sweater and pushed her head under the dishwater in the sink. That was all the fight I had in me and I started shaking all over. I was scared of what she would do to me and what the matrons would do, but mostly I was scared of my own anger.

The girl didn't tell on me and all the girls were nicer to me after that. The girl I had nearly drowned and I became close friends. She was from a cattle ranch in the south eastern part of Montana and although she came from a good family, she got involved with a wild crowd and started drinking when she went to high school in Billings. She was with two boys one night when they stole some beer from a gas station and they had a gun in the car when they were stopped by the police.

She had cigarettes in her room and when we smoked upstairs we blew the smoke out of the screened windows. She asked me once if I really would have drowned her and I told her I wasn't sure. I explained that I had never been in a fight before and I didn't do what I did on purpose; it just happened.

"God," she said. "You might be dangerous. What if you couldn't stop?"

"I don't know," I admitted to her and to myself.

I learned that my dad was going back to Alaska when I stumbled on a story in the Great Falls Tribune. He and seven other people, who the article referred to as Argonauts, had left for an area 150 miles south of Fairbanks. They planned to develop a 40,000 acre cattle spread. There were photos of some of the families that were staying behind, the huge caravan of trucks and combines, and of my dad—who said he had nothing to lose—holding his skillet. I remembered my mother's words. "He just uses her to bring attention to himself." I felt like he had figured out how to get attention without me and for awhile I hated my dad but I guess I was using him when I showed the girls the newspaper story and the picture of my dad holding his skillet.

I did well in my studies that spring. There were only seven students in some of my classes and the individual attention given to me by the teachers was just what I needed to renew my love of learning.

When the school year ended, the girls who had been there more than six months could go home for one week. They went home to parents, grandparents or other relatives. I didn't get to leave and neither did Loretta so we chummed around and learned to play canasta.

I learned something else that summer. We went into town for swimming sessions at the YWCA and played soft ball against the Helena teams. The softball coach, a young athletically attractive woman, was alive with energy and enthusiasm. I was drawn to her in a way I didn't understand. I convinced the administrator that it would be a learning experience for me to be an assistant softball coach. I was given extra privileges such as staying off campus late for in-town games and riding in the coach's car. Of course the girls were jealous of my preferential treatment and one day one of the Indian girls called me a queer. After that the others made hateful remarks about me and the coach. They said I was becoming a lesbian because I acted like I was in love with the coach. I did have feelings for her that I didn't understand. I felt almost dizzy in her presence and I blushed when she spoke to me. Just sitting in her car by myself made me feel good all over, but I didn't think I was queer. There were girls in the school who did experiment with each other by kissing and fondling and I found that behavior disgusting. One night I walked to Miss Tallman's resident room and when she asked me what I needed, I wanted to ask her to hold me, but I didn't. She took me back to the dorm area and she told Miss Susan I seemed upset about something.

I didn't get to be an assistant coach after that and the coach avoided me. I couldn't understand why she had turned on me and I was very sad when she went home for her summer break. She didn't come back in the fall and that was my only brush with lesbianism.

Some nonsense was tolerated by the staff but occasionally the girls went too far. One morning my friend came down the stairs wearing a state dress that had a small hole in it. I playfully put my finger in the hole and ripped the dress off of her—which was something all of us did at least once. Unfortunately for me, Miss Vagina was coming down the hall at that very moment. She grabbed me and literally pulled me by my hair across the campus to the main building. Miss Miller slapped my bare legs several times with a wooden starch paddle that left welts meant to be a warning to the others.

Another thing we did, that got a bunch of us in trouble, was decorate the jail cell in the basement. I don't think anyone was ever put in that old dungeon room, but several of us risk takers decided to make the cell comfortable, just in case. We tugged an old davenport in there and put a rug on the floor. With a nice floor lamp, a few pillows and some makeshift curtains it became a nice little nest for any of us that might be locked in there. Not long after our interior decorating was completed the night watch matron woke us up at 4am and told us to have the cell cleaned out before breakfast.

There were frequent runners and attempts at running and the best route was out the kitchen door and across the open fields toward the Sleeping Giant mountain north of the school. After dark, we would watch as the lights from the patrol cars searched the hills. I wanted to run away and have someone run after me and force me to come back, but when I did pretend I was going to run, Miss Susan hollered at me to get back in the cottage before I got in trouble; she went in without looking to see if I was coming back. I did.

We frequently went to Lake Hauser to swim and picnic and in August the entire school went to Yellowstone Park for a week. We rode a tour bus and unloaded tents and camping equipment every night. Before school started I got to leave for a week. I went to Grandma's in Great Falls and was surprised how shoddy our one room home seemed. My friends had formed new cliques and I was odd man out.

Because I had failed almost all of my classes at Great Falls High while I was trying to get married, I didn't have any credits toward my graduation. I started high school over and discovered I loved math and science. I pecked around on the piano, drums, saxophone and clarinet and I sang alto in the choir. I made a paper Mache' skunk in art class that Miss Miller put on display in the administration building. I joined the speech and debate team and decided to try for membership in the National Thespian Society. I needed a leading role in a drama production to get enough points for membership. I tried out for a part in a minstrel show as a black girl and I got the part. I liked being someone other than myself. I could become the character without fear of what others say about me because I was acting. It wasn't really me. In November the parts for the school's annual Christmas program that was performed on stage in Helena were posted on the bulletin board. The story was about a crippled boy who came to the manger. I wanted that part so bad that I cut off my long auburn hair and dyed it black. I practiced limping around with one crutch so everyone would remember I wanted the part.

My friend came running into the math classroom to let me know I had the part. "Carol! You got it. You got it. You get to be the shepard boy!" she gushed. "You just have to call your Dad and tell him to come to see you in the play."

Dad was back in Montana. He didn't stay in Alaska once the equipment was unloaded and a kitchen set up for the homesteaders. He called and said he was working in Sweet Grass, a tiny town on the Canadian Border. He told me I would be able to spend Christmas break with him up there. He had kept a journal and taken a lot pictures on the trek to Alaska and was anxious to show me. He even talked about the two of us going back to Alaska when I got out of the school. I called him and asked him to come and watch the play. He said he would make it a point to be there and that then I could ride with him to Sweet Grass for the holiday.

That was about two weeks before the performance. I didn't hear from him any more before opening night. I thought perhaps he had gone straight to the theater instead of stopping at the school so as I made my way down the center aisle on the crutch, I looked for him in the crowd. The lights were low, it was hard to see, and then once I was on stage the spotlights made it impossible to see out into the audience. I played my heart out to my father who I believed was out there applauding me.

After the third curtain call, while we were changing into our regular clothes, Miss Miller told me she was so sorry to tell me that my dad had not made it to Helena. He had called from Great Falls and because it was snowing hard in the mountains, I was to catch the bus the next day and meet him in Great Falls. At the cast party that evening I wondered if it had been a whiskey bottle and a card game instead of the snow that had kept my dad from getting to Helena.

Dad met me in Great Falls and we had dinner with Grandma before leaving for Sweet Grass. He was the Black Jack dealer in a nightclub owned by a family named Fontaine. Mrs. Fontaine, Vi, was a middle-aged woman with short auburn hair who wore silk dressing gowns in private and saddle pants and sweaters when she was working. She always used a long cigarette holder when she smoked. Her husband, Lynn, was not really a big man; but he swaggered around the place to make sure everyone, including the women, knew that he was the boss. Joyce, Vi's daughter from a previous marriage, had a little boy named Ricky. People said the boy belonged to Lynn. Vi had sent Joyce away to have the baby and when she came back, she said they had adopted a baby boy."

I had a nice Christmas in Sweet Grass. Vi treated me like a special guest and made sure there were gifts under their tree for me. I especially enjoyed playing with Joyce's little boy. Joyce was friendly, but very quiet. She seemed to curl inward when she sat as well as when she walked. Not only was she small, she was mousy in her mannerisms and her appearance. She wore rimless glasses that showed the full width of her too wide face and her high forehead.

I thought Lynn was very handsome. He had square shoulders and slim hips. When he walked his pelvis led the way. He combed his dark hair to one side and he could have been mistaken for a movie idol. But when he smiled his thin lips stretched across his teeth in a sinister way.

Lynn, Vi and Joyce all worked in the bar at night and had an apartment behind the dance hall. The nightclub, which also had a restaurant and some gaming tables, had live music on weekends and I listened to the music and bar crowd while I babysat Ricky in the back.

When I returned to Sweet Grass for spring break Vi asked me if I would like to work for them as a nanny for Ricky. She said they would pay all of my school expenses and give me an allowance. I agreed and Vi called the school to make arrangements.

In June of 1954 I jumped from the frying pan into the fire.

CHAPTER 9—SWEET GRASS

My stay in Sweet Grass would be a journey of betrayal that would stretch across four seasons. I settled into the high-back seat in the bus that would carry me to yet another uncertain future with mixed feelings. On one hand, I had experienced some security at the reform school. I had lived comfortably behind locked doors and barred windows and had made strides in my academic growth and personal development, on the other hand, the opportunity for me to learn an acceptable way to navigate through my teen years without a mother was presenting itself. I was also worried about my relationship with my dad who might not know how to relate to the changes in his tomboy daughter.

The interstate highway ends at Sweet Grass where citizens checked through customs at the international border. Some houses in the town sat on the border and their front porch was in the United States while their back yard was in Canada. About one hundred and fifty people lived in Sweet Grass, Montana and Coutts, Alberta. They were hardy individuals, who tolerated isolation caused by distance and weather. Like other farm communities scattered across the Golden Triangle of North Central Montana, there was a couple of clapboard hotels and twice that many taverns. The post office, a farm implement shop, and a general mercantile store met the immediate needs of the town people between shopping trips to Great Falls that was one hundred and thirty miles to the south. Farmers trucked their grain seven miles south to the elevators in Sunburst and when the children graduated from the two-room schoolhouse on the edge of town, they were bused to Sunburst

Union High School. A few families lived in the weathered houses on the town's half dozen arterial streets, but many of the structures had been abandoned. Merchant's depended on the surrounding farmers for business.

To the west, across the checkerboard grain fields and past grasslands that butted up to the Rocky Mountain front, the continental divide separates cowboy Montana from logger Montana. Montana's eastern flatlands challenge individuals to be tough, determined and rugged, but reveals her fickle temperament with brilliant sunsets over purple thrusts of magnificent mountains. Summer winds caress tired cowboys at the end of a roundup and Chinooks roaring across wintered lands provides relief from subzero temperatures until the next blizzard slams down from the north. In all directions, as far as the eye can see, the big sky of Montana sits down upon the earth. The cone-shaped Sweet Grass Hills, thirty miles east, look like pyramids as the sun begins to light the sky behind them.

That day, traveling northward from Great Falls, the pastures and prairies were soft with spring grasses waving in the breeze. I searched the bleached shorelines of alkali ponds for mallards or Canadian geese. I wondered if my dad would remember to meet the bus.   He was there, like he had promised. He hugged me hard and called me kiddo and I felt like I was back in the Montana that I loved. The little house on the main street that he had rented was once a gift shop. The display windows were painted part way up to provide privacy and allow light into the two-room house. There was a kitchen with a day bed, which would be mine, a bedroom, and a tiny bathroom. My dad had another roommate; a rhesus monkey named Bimbo. Dad said if he rolled on Bimbo during the night the monkey would scream so I shouldn't be alarmed if I heard a commotion. The monkey was dirty, mean and disgusting, and I was glad when my dad moved him to a cage in the night club. Bimbo was a conversation piece for the bar customers, but he caused the Fontaine women a great deal of embarrassment because he was able to do what the rock star who had a rib removed couldn't. Lynn and Clint, the bartender, threw Tabasco sauce on the monkey to make him stop pleasuring himself. Bimbo would then jump up and down in the cage screaming and showing his teeth, his round eyes bulging in his face. They were never sure if he was mad about the stinging sauce or because he was interrupted.

My first day back in Sweetgrass went quickly. After I put my things away, Dad and I walked up the street. We stopped in a couple of taverns where he introduced me to people he knew. According to Daddy the holes in the glass bricks surrounding the entrance to the Fontaines' place were bullet holes. The large dance floor between the bar and the family's private quarters had built-in leather booths on two sides; at one end of the dance floor there was a small stage with a piano and a set of drums. A lunch counter and several dining tables were in the restaurant-side of the establishment. A gaming area had one round poker table and a horseshoe-shaped blackjack table. My dad was the blackjack dealer.

Vi explained what my job would be. Besides taking care of the little boy I would work in the café sometimes. In exchange my school expenses and spending money would be provided. She said I could help myself to soda pop and cigarettes, and eat anything in the café. Ricky, who was by then a one-year-old, was a chubby little guy with a happy smile. I looked forward to spending time with him. Joyce worked in the nightclub on busy nights. The living room had a crib for Ricky and a hide-a-bed, where I could sleep until she finished working. Lynn slept in the hide-a-bed and Joyce slept with her mother in the bedroom.

I enjoyed the summer. Ricky was just beginning to walk and I followed him around the dance floor or pulled him around town in his wagon. Dad worked until the nightclub closed, so I walked home with him each night. Vi, joking around, introduced me to people as her new daughter and I hoped she meant it. Lynn teased me about the reform school and Whitey, and although I didn't like the comments he made, I liked the attention. Clint, their bartender, had black curly hair and wore black-rimmed glasses. He looked more like a professor or a banker than a bartender. He wore a white shirt and a bow tie while he was working. He filled me in on the history of the people in Sweet Grass, as well as that of the Fontaine family. He said the holes in the glass bricks really were bullet holes, but they weren't the result of a western-type shootout. They had come from inside the nightclub when Lynn, in a drunken rage one night, fired his gun at them. Clint also told me that when Joyce got pregnant, Vi sent her to a home for unwed mothers. Vi told everyone that Joyce was going to business school in Great Falls. When Joyce came back to Sweet Grass with a baby, she said that they had adopted the little boy. Clint said no one in town believed that story. When I asked Daddy if he knew about Ricky, he said everyone did, and added that Vi was either a fool or a saint.

I became friends with Donna, who was my age; we both worked in the cafe. She had a horse, and she knew people who would let me ride their horse. When we weren't working, we walked a mile east of town to the pasture where the horses were, and spent a lot of time shaking oats in a can to catch them. We rode bareback, and Lynn teased us about getting our "rocks off" while we were riding; he said that our jeans weren't wet from sweating. When we told him he was gross he just threw his head back and laughed at us.

Once a month someone from the bar had to travel to Great Falls for supplies. If we all went, I was expected to be in charge of Ricky. I enjoyed those trips because we stayed at the opulent Park Hotel with its red carpeting and bell boys dressed in military-type uniforms. With a list of items to purchase for Ricky, I pushed him around town in the stroller and pretended he was mine. When I took him over to Grandma's she laughed about my job. She said I was getting paid to play with dolls.

The family was on vacation at Flathead Lake when something happened that scared me. Joyce and I were sitting in the car with Ricky waiting for Lynn and Vi to come out of a tavern. Joyce asked me to go in and see if I could get them to leave so we could go back to the motel. Lynn was at the bar talking with a couple of men and when I interrupted him he said, "Oh, my women are after me; they sent the young one."

He reached out and pinched my breast. I playfully kicked him in the shin, and he just laughed. When we got back to the motel he showed Vi where I had kicked him. Vi asked, "Did you really do that?"

When I told her I was just playing around, she said I was lucky he didn't come back at me with a fist.

I told Clint what had happened while we gone on vacation, and about what Vi said. He said she was probably right. Then he told me one time Vi had been standing behind the bar washing glasses and she said something that Lynn didn't like. According to Clint's story, Lynn had vaulted over the bar with one hand and knocked her down with the other before Vi could even duck.

"You better be careful around Lynn if you know what's good for you," he warned.

I learned to make donuts using the deep fat fryer in the café. They were good donuts, and before long they were selling as fast as I could make them. After I paid for the ingredients, I made a nice profit.

One evening, while I was in the pantry washing dishes, Lynn came in and rubbed his front against my butt. When I pulled away, he slipped his finger under my bra strap and told me it was dirty.

"I want you to wear a clean bra every day," he ordered.

I was afraid of him but I found my pulse racing when he was near me or when he said something personal to me. I liked to watch him, but I didn't want him to know that.

One night when I walked home from work with Dad he was slurring his words. I began to get ready for bed and he called me into his room and asked me if he could look at my breasts. I was frightened. I said no and told him to go to bed. He kept on pleading with me, saying that he want to see if I was growing into a woman. I argued with him for over an hour before he passed out. The next morning I told Vi I wanted to move out of my dad's place; I told her why. She rented a room for me about a block from the night club. That afternoon while I was packing my things, Dad kept apologizing; saying he had been drinking. He said he didn't remember anything after we got home that night. I said it didn't matter what he remembered.

"I remember and I'm leaving before you rape me like you did my sister."

At first he angrily denied doing anything to Margaret, and then he began ranting that I would get pregnant like Joyce and if that happened he was going to cut Lynn's balls off. I left while he was cussing and yelling at me. After that when I saw him around town I thought he looked sad and although I felt bad about what happened, I didn't speak to him.

The next time Lynn went to Great Falls for supplies, he asked Jim, the poker dealer to go with him, and he asked me if I wanted to ride along to visit my grandma. I sat in the front seat between the two men and pretended to be asleep. I leaned against Lynn who was driving. We checked into three separate rooms at the Park Hotel but when I heard a key in my door I knew it would be Lynn. I started to say something but he shushed me whispering that Jim might have heard him coming into my room. I welcomed his advances as he climbed into my bed, but I was surprised at the pain that came with my first real experience with intercourse. I think Lynn was surprised that it was my first time. I guess Whitey had just rubbed around on me. Lynn left the room as soon as he was done without saying anything. There were many more times that we were together like that. When Joyce and Vi were working in the nightclub he locked the apartment door and quickly did his thing. It was his thing. I had no role other than to lie still and be quiet. It didn't bother me that he never kissed me, because I thought it was obvious that he couldn't resist me, and I was madly in love. I enjoyed having that secret between my lover and me. Whenever our eyes met in the bar or the restaurant, I felt my heart skip a beat.

I celebrated my sixteenth birthday at a grange hall dance in Alberta. The kids in Sweet Grass crammed into one car and shared the gas expense to drive to those dances every weekend. I learned to dance and I learned to sip from the bottles in paper sacks passed around the parking lot, but I never went further than a kiss with the boys I danced with. My heart belonged to a real man.

When I started high school in Sunburst, I discovered I had enough credits to skip my sophomore year. I had to take two English classes to meet the graduation requirements, but I enrolled as a junior. Kids gathered at the farm implement store each morning to catch the bus and I usually slept on the way to school because I had worked late. I did my homework at night after I put Ricky to bed. Thanks to my donut business I had angora socks that matched my sweaters. Each morning I stopped at the bar for some lunch money and a package of cigarettes. I got along with the kids at school, and even began going to football games and other activities.

Donna and I were working in the café when we got into an argument over who was going to use the deep fat fryer. I wanted to make some donuts before she used the new grease for chicken or French fries. We were behind the counter and screaming at each other when Lynn walked in. He came up to me and without any warning brought his fist under my jaw so hard my feet came off the floor.

"Don't ever let me catch you harassing my hired help again," he said.

He turned and walked out of the café and I couldn't believe he could do that to me. I was embarrassed, but I couldn't open my mouth to say anything. Donna rushed over and put her arm around me trying to console me, but I shook her off and ran out of the café and away from the customers that were staring at me. I had to drink through a straw for a few days, but my jaw wasn't broken, only my heart. When Lynn approached me for sex a short time after that I lied and said I had my period but I didn't.

My period, which was very regular, didn't come around at all in December, I knew when I started back to school that I might be pregnant. Each time I went to the bathroom I checked my panties; I began hoping that I was going to have a baby. After missing my period the second time I made up excuses for not participating in the more strenuous gym activities, and by the first part of March I quit going to the gym classes.

Donna and I traveled to Great Falls for the class AA basketball tournament. I stayed with Margaret, and I went to a couple of basketball games before I told Donna I thought I was pregnant. I picked a doctor listed in the phone book, and Donna went with me to the appointment. She sat in the waiting room while I went in with the nurse. Dr. Keenan laughed when I suggested I might have a tumor. He I should start thinking about a name for the tumor, but then he talked with me about my options. In 1955 Hollywood stars were not showing off their babies before marriage. Unwed mothers went to homes where they were encouraged to give up their babies. Although abortions did happen, I was almost four months along, too late for that. The nurse gave me some literature to take home and suggested I think about what would be best for the baby. I walked back into the waiting room carrying the pamphlets and when Donna saw them she screamed, "O my God! Carol, what are you going to do?"

I grabbed her sleeve and pulled her out of there as quick as I could. I made her swear to keep my secret. I told her I didn't know who the father was. I didn't tell my sister I was pregnant and it was a long time before anyone found out.

Clint and Joyce figured it out at about the same time. Clint was a bachelor, as far as I knew anyway. I asked him, in just a conversational way, if he would marry a person who was pregnant and didn't have anywhere to turn. He laughed and said there was no way he would settle into a marriage of convenience with someone else's baby. I guess he suspected I had a personal reason for asking him that question, and he told Joyce. She put two and two together when she walked into the bathroom while I was bathing, and noticed my swollen breasts and round abdomen. She asked me when I was due. I was five months along when Vi and Joyce sat me down to talk. Vi thought maybe I could wear a girdle and finish the school year, but Joyce pleaded with her mother not to do that to me. They asked me who the baby's father was so many times that I began crying. Lynn told them to leave me alone. He said, "How could she know who the father was when she slept with every boy in the area?"

They decided that I could continue working for them, and that I would go to school as long as I could. Pregnant girls were not allowed to attend school and by the first part of May the principal called me into his office. He said he really hated to ask me to drop out because I had top grades, even taking two years in one, but he had no choice. He made arrangements for me to study at home, and he said I could return for finals. Donna collected my assignments and returned them to the teachers for me; and I finished my junior year. I even purchased the class ring, ruby and mother-of-pearl, our class colors.

By June everyone in town knew I was pregnant, and my dad had no doubt about whom the father of the baby was. Once, when we met on the sidewalk, he told me he was going to castrate Lynn, but that's all he ever said to me about it. I don't think he even told Lynn what he thought. There wasn't DNA testing back then, but Lynn could have faced a jail sentence for statutory rape. I loyally denied knowing who the baby's father was.

Clint said he was sorry he wasn't able to help me. He told me some day I would understand. That day may have come sooner than he intended. He had been dating an unattractive older woman for a couple of years. People in town made jokes about Mabel's crush on Clint. Her obese body was found in her house on the outskirts of town hacked to pieces. No one knew how long she had been dead, but shortly after that

Clint was taken into custody. Clint was cleared of any charges, but he didn't return to Sweetgrass.

My dad got into a similar situation early that summer. Donna and I were working in the café when we heard a commotion in the nightclub. An Indian man came running through the door. Blood gushing out of the side of his head splattered the counter as he ran out of the café and crossed the street with my dad—holding a hammer in the air—right behind him. They ran between buildings across the street before my dad gave up the chase. Dad had accused the Indian, who had been playing cards, of cheating. The Indian pulled out a knife and held it at my dad's throat. Somehow my dad had twisted out of the knife's way, and grabbed a hammer from under the table and hit the Indian in the head. The only law enforcement, the sheriff forty miles away in Shelby, never came and we never knew what happened to the cheating Indian.

I found an antique iron crib and painted it white. Donna's mother gave me a baby shower and I had everything I needed for a newborn. What I didn't have was a clue what to do with a baby. I foolishly thought I could bring the baby back to Sweet Grass and continue life as it was.

Before my seventeenth birthday Vi told me I would be going to Great Falls to stay until the baby was born. She had called my sister, but Margaret didn't want her children to see me or know anything about the baby. Vi called the Columbus Hospital and the Sisters of Charity agreed I could stay there and work off my hospital bill before the baby was born. We stopped in Shelby and Joyce bought me a cute maternity outfit for my birthday. I met with the Sister in charge of the maternity ward and she showed me the room where I could stay until my baby came. I walked back out to the car with Joyce and Vi to say goodbye, and when he pulled away from the curb, Lynn tooted the horn.

I worked four hours each morning rolling gauze balls and making maternity packets. I had the rest of the day to myself. I ate most of my meals at the hospital and I spent a lot of time in town with Grandma. Margaret called the hospital to let me know she would be with me when my time came.

Sometimes at night I heard terrible screams before one of the nuns rushed down the hall and closed my door.

I went to the state fair on the eighth of August. Like my mother, I loved the fair. Even though my ankles were swollen and my back ached

I planned to go to the fair again the next day. I had a bad back ache the next morning, so I asked for some pills. The nurse she said maybe she should check me; I had already dilated to five centimeters. I was in labor! She said she thought my baby would be born that evening so I called Margaret to tell her I was in labor, but that she didn't need to come to the hospital until after work. I walked around rubbing my back until I told Sister it was worse. She put me in the labor room and called Margaret. By the time my sister arrived, about 1:30 p.m., I was in hard labor and soon delivered a tiny baby boy. Gardner Dean Johnson weighed five pounds, nine ounces, and was eighteen inches long.

That evening, August 9, I watched the sunset. The clouds turned a cotton candy pink. I thought of the fair and my mother and wondered about the miracle of life. I couldn't believe I was a mother and the experience touched me so deeply that tears of wonder fall silently down my cheeks. I had a baby. He was mine! No one could take him away from me! I wasn't alone anymore.

CHAPTER 10—GARDNER

"What do you want his birth certificate for? So he can find out he's illegitimate someday?" the nurse at the desk snarled at me. Several nuns had approached me about giving my baby up for adoption, but in my mind it was not an option. The baby was my family.

"I just want the one with his footprints on it for a souvenir, that's all." I explained.

Gardner was perfect from his fuzzy head to his tiny toes. He was small, chubby in all the right places. He had little fat wrinkles behind his knees and on his wrists and even a little under his quivering chin. I had to leave the hospital after the usual five day stay. I didn't have a plan but I knew that I could go to Grandma's. I had spent the last of my trust fund money for a crib and some other baby items. On the fourth day one of the nurses said I could live with her and her husband. I moved into their extra bedroom in the motel they called home and the next week I went to work as a housekeeper for the hospital. I cleaned bathrooms, dusted the floors, and put fresh water in flower vases. I went to work at 7 a.m. and got off at 3:30 p.m. just as my friend was coming on for the afternoon shift. She brought my baby with her; and then I rode back to the motel with her husband. When Gardner was three weeks old, the nurse got caught stealing drugs, so I had to go to Grandma's after all. The baby and I, his crib, diaper pails, and all the sterilization equipment moved into her dirty one-room apartment on a stifling hot August day. What I knew about babies I learned in a book. I believed everything that touched the baby had to be sterile and nothing in that brownstone, including my grandma, was. I didn't know then that love can't be boiled or sanitized.

Making enough baby formula for one day was a lot like canning peaches and Gardner's diapers were cloth. They had to be soaked, washed (sometimes boiled), and preferably dried in the sun. Grandma's little corner sink and the drunks' bathtub down the hall were the only place I could do the laundry, and when I used the stove to make the formula the temperature in Grandma's room was intolerable.

Grandma wanted me to go to Kellogg, Idaho where Uncle Ralph and Aunt Lucille lived. We rode a Greyhound bus all night and most of the next day before we reached the border of Montana. Lookout Pass was a winding narrow road that clung to the side of the mountain high above a colorful valley below. Golden aspens and yellow birch leaves winked through white-barked trees as they welcomed autumn.

Uncle Ralph and Aunt Lucille lived on a small acreage at the edge of town with a few animals. Uncle Ralph's geese followed him when he walked to town to get the mail, and then followed him back home. Cats and dogs lazed in the warm sun that afternoon when Uncle Ralph turned into the driveway with Grandma, the baby, and me, all sitting in the front of his old pickup truck. Aunt Lucille let the screen door slam as she rushed out to greet us. She hugged us and then took Gardner from me. "O, Carol, he is just perfect," she crooned as she pressed her face to his.

Grandma stayed a couple of weeks before we took her back to the bus. I packed my little bundle around downtown Kellogg, applying for jobs with no success. On the days I didn't go to town I slept on my bed with the baby near me. I was homesick and worried. Ralph and Lucille wanted to adopt Gardner, and I wasn't sure I could stop them from doing that.

They insisted that I attend the Assembly of God church with them. I didn't mind going to church, but this one was much different from my Catholic experiences. Everyone knelt on the floor to pray with their heads bowed in the pew and they prayed out loud in "tongues." Every Sunday and Wednesday evening, too, people knelt around me and prayed for me to give my heart to the Lord. I didn't want forgiveness for having the baby that I loved and I loved Lynn too. I didn't want them, or God, to think I was ashamed of that love but I didn't want them to force me to give Gardner to my aunt and uncle so when they prayed, I cried, and while they rocked and moaned I said the words they wanted to hear.

Dad called to tell us that Grandma had died. Lucille called the hospital to find out what had happened, and a nurse told her Grandma had died peacefully. She had been in the nursing home for about a month with kidney failure. Lucille was worried about Grandma's soul but according to the nurse at the nursing home Grandma had turned to the Lord before she died. I always wondered if Lucille made that part up. Grandma was sixty-eight when she died. When I was seventeen, I thought that was long enough to live anyway.

We all traveled to Great Falls to join the rest of the family for Grandma's funeral at Croxford's. She was buried in Highland Cemetery near her youngest child, and not far from my mother's grave. I felt like the last safety net in my life was gone.

I turned to the Fontaines for help. While I was in Idaho, Joyce and Lynn had left Sweet Grass and started a home of their own in Great Falls. Joyce was expecting another baby. Gardner and I stayed at with them until I got a nanny job. I got fired from that job because I cleaned the house. The husband made such a big deal about the house being clean his wife got mad and told me she hired me to take care of her children, not to clean.

I went back to the Fontaine's with the baby and each morning after the Thanksgiving holiday, I wrapped Gardner in heavy blankets and took the bus into town to look for a job. Some people said they didn't have any openings, but others offered me a chance to warm up in their break room, or gave me a cup of coffee while I filled out the paper work.

One time, Lynn told me it was a good thing the baby looked like me or he would have had to throw both of us into the river. I believed he would do that. When we were all living in Sweet Grass, he had made Vi, Joyce, and me stand against a wall while he pointed a gun at each of us and I heard rumors that he had connections with the Mafia in Great Falls. The only time he offered to help me with my baby was once when Gardner had diarrhea and Lynn drove me to the doctor and gave me some money to pay the bill. Later, he drove to a secluded spot in the country. I told him no. I said, "You have never even kissed me.

Here I am the mother of your son you don't care about me at all, so I don't want to have sex with you anymore."

Lynn laughed and threw back his head "Hell, all you ever had to do was say no. I thought you liked it. I sure ain't going to rape you."

Had it really been my own fault? I never liked the sex part, but I did want him to love me.

Joyce was concerned that I was dragging the baby around town in subzero weather; she suggested I try to get on welfare. I left Gardner with her one day and went to apply for assistance. I was nervous about getting involved with the state. The welfare office was in the basement of the courthouse, in the same building as the office of the judge who had sent me to Helena. But I found I could get financial help, and before Christmas Gardner and I had our own place to live; two rooms in the basement of a three-story apartment building. I put Gardner's crib in the bedroom, and laid out the materials I used to sterilize his formula on the Formica countertop. Joyce helped me get a few dishes and some bedding at the Salvation Army store. I got $90 a month from which I paid $45 for rent.

I bathed my baby in the kitchen sink every night, polished his tiny shoes, and followed the instructions from a baby-care book religiously. If Gardner was hungry before the scheduled time, he had to wait, no matter how hard he cried. I found a used stroller with a fiddle-shaped metal seat. He couldn't sit up alone, so I propped him against the back of the stroller with a pillow and took him out for the scheduled 10 a.m. airing, no matter what the temperature was. Irma, the landlady who lived on the main floor watched me lug the stroller outside one day and said, "I'm afraid you are either going to break that baby's neck, or freeze him to death."

I explained that I was following the instructions in a baby-care book and she just clucked her tongue and went back into her apartment.

There were no instructions in the book about when and how to hug or cuddle. Fortunately Mother Nature knows that socialization is critical to human development, and Gardner began smiling and cooing which causing me to interact with him at unscheduled times. He grew a ring of auburn colored hair around his bald head, and his chubby-cheeked smile charmed people who stopped to coo over him.

In December, I spent the entire welfare check at Public Drugs for Christmas decorations and gifts. Irma's husband cut down a Christmas tree for his family and brought one for me too. When the Salvation Army called to tell me that someone had turned my name in for a holiday basket, I assured them that I had everything I needed. I opened a charge account at the grocery store where Grandma used to shop. The next month, after I paid the rent and the grocery bill, I had about five dollars left to spend.

Margaret came to see me during the holidays, and brought some gifts to put under my tree. While she was there she handed me a gold band to wear as a wedding ring. She said she told Diane and Gary, and the people she worked with at Woolworths, that I had married a soldier boy who was overseas. She explained that she had told them the reason the birth announcement hadn't been in the paper was because the baby weighed less than five pounds—in 1955, illegitimate births and premature babies who might not live were not listed in the paper—then she invited us to come to their house for Christmas dinner.

I enjoyed showing the baby to my niece and nephew, and he squealed with delight when they played with him. Margaret cooked a nice dinner and carried Gardner around, cooing at him and telling me what a doll he was. Walt even held him for a little while. It was a good day and I wore the ring every day after that.

By February I had found a real husband in the military. Bill Gordon was a nineteen-year-old flyboy from Redding California. I met him at a party, and he started coming over to my apartment. He seemed to enjoy helping with Gardner, and sometimes brought groceries so I could make us something to eat. Bill was handsome with sharp features and very black hair. We were married in the Malmstrom Air Force Base chapel. The couple who lived across the hall from me stood up for us. Margaret didn't come. She said she was afraid it would confuse her children. The last time I had seen Dad I had stopped in the Club Cigar store with the baby. Dad bought me a hamburger, and told me I had ruined my future. He said Gardner was a "cute little bastard." So I didn't invite my dad to the wedding or to the party in the bowling alley that my friends in the apartment held for Bill and me.

About six weeks after the wedding and the party—six weeks after the gifts had all been opened and used—I told Bill I didn't like being married. He said he didn't either, so we decided not to be. I packed his things for him, and he took them when he left for work that morning. I saw him one more time. He came in the afternoon and knocked on what used to be our door, but was now my door. He said I forgot to pack his alarm clock. He waited in the hall, and when I handed him the clock he asked if we were supposed to kiss goodbye. I told him I didn't think so. That was the last time I ever saw my first husband. I received papers from him confirming an annulment two years later.

Irma, the landlady, and her husband had an adopted daughter who was married and lived on the upper floor of the building. Thelma was pregnant when I first became friends with her. Her mother was worried about the pregnancy because Thelma had been bedridden as a child with rheumatic fever. She was still thin, pale and tired easily. She got pregnant against her doctor's advice. Even her husband had pleaded with her not to try to have a child. She spent a lot of time in bed conserving her strength so she could be up when Rolph came home for supper. I spent afternoons with her. After I settled Gardner into a playpen for his nap, Thelma and I played cards, looked at books with baby names, chose recipes to try, or just talked about girlfriends things. Thelma was afraid that she might not be able to have the baby and she asked a lot of questions about the birth process. On Saturday night the two of us joined others from the building who gathered in the apartment across the hall from me. Those neighbors had a television and invited everyone to watch The Lawrence Welk Show.

I got a phone call from Joyce me one day. She and Lynn wanted to talk to me about something and Lynn was on his way to pick me up. I was surprised to hear from them. I hadn't seen them since before my short-lived marriage. Joyce was waiting for me in the living room. When I sat down, Lynn looked me in the eye and said, "What in the hell is going on. Your landlady told us you are telling people that baby is mine?"

Before I could answer, Joyce added, "My God, Carol, how do you think that makes me look? After all I've done for you. I can't believe that you are telling people something like that."

Lynn glared at me as he added, "Don't you realize I could go to prison for messing around with someone your age? We have tried to be family and this is the kind of thanks we get?"

"This is so embarrassing Carol. Why would you do this to us?" Joyce questioned.

I was struck speechless by the surprise attack and by the way that Lynn feigned his innocence and indignation.

"I don't know," I whispered.

"Is that all you have to say, for Christ's sake!" stormed Lynn.

"I'm sorry I told people that," I offered.

I liked Joyce and I didn't want her to know the truth. I didn't want her to dislike me, and I didn't want her to know that her husband was a liar. I was scared that Lynn might do something to Gardner and me. I sat on their couch with my baby and wished I could melt away. I said I would tell Irma and Thelma that I had been lying. Lynn took me back to the apartment and he said I better keep my mouth shut if I knew what was good for me. I didn't see either Lynn or Joyce until June when she had Michael. I took her a gift while she was in the hospital. Thelma had a baby boy too. She named him Darwin, after her dad. Gardner learned how to crawl out of his crib and playpen and one day I found him half a block away crossing a street in his draw-string nightgown.

One day Uncle Ralph called me from a hotel downtown. He asked me if I wanted to ride with them to the funeral the next day. I didn't even know that Uncle Toppy had died. On the way to the funeral home, Aunt Lucille told me that Uncle Joe had committed suicide shortly after Grandma died and that Edith had finally died from the tuberculosis she had fought so many years. It seemed like all of my family was dying. Gardner wasn't even a year old, and four people had died since he was born. My cousins were in the family room at Croxford's when we arrived. I didn't see them until we were at the cemetery. I went up to them and hugged them and we cried together. Dad was there too, and when he hugged me I felt, for a short time that day, like we were family again.

Not long after that funeral, Aunt Lucille called from Idaho to tell me that Uncle Ralph had a brain tumor.

While my family circle was getting smaller, new friends were filling in the vacant spaces and soon I would have a family of my own. On the Fourth, Irma had a picnic for all the tenants. Everybody brought potluck items to Gibson Park and we sat on blankets or folding chairs to watch the fireworks. Gardner crawled around in the grass and Thelma nursed her baby boy under a blanket over her shoulder. A little boy and girl who came to the apartment sometimes to stay with their dad who lived on the main floor were at the picnic too. That day as his children played on the swings their father asked me how old Gardner was. He told me he was a flight engineer, and worked out at the base refueling planes in the air. When he asked about my husband, having heard that he was in the Air Force too, I told him I was divorced. He told me his children, Patty and Danny, lived at St. Thomas Orphanage most of the time and he was surprised to hear that I had lived there too. He said their mother kept the youngest boy, David, and he took the older children. We ate together and talked all that day, getting to know a lot about each other before the fireworks started.

After that, whenever Patty was staying with her dad, he sent her down to my apartment so I could comb her long, brown hair. It was hard for me to get the tangles out without hurting her, and she always wound up crying. She hated living at St. Thomas and she didn't like living with her dad either. She wanted to live with her mother. She said she liked playing with Gardner, but she missed her little brother. Danny avoided me even when we all went out for a hamburger or to a drive-in movie. He seemed shy and stayed in his dad's room drawing pictures or listening to the radio. Dan sat on the front porch visiting with the other tenets on his days off and he seemed to fit into our apartment "family" very well. I was attracted to him and tried to flirt, but he gave me a dime and told me to call him on my eighteenth birthday. He was thirty-four.

On the nineteenth of July, I called him and he took me to the Cub's Den in Monarch and a drive-in movie. Dan was the richest man I had ever met. He had a brand new car, and he made over $350 a month. In August, when Gardner had his birthday party, Dan took us to town with his children and bought complete outfits for all of us and some toys for Gardner.

Before school started in September, Dan took his children out of the orphanage, and we moved into a two-bedroom place and decided to be a family.

CHAPTER 11—THE BANICH FAMILY

My personal journey brought me from a unique childhood where I had strived to make sense out of my personal realities, into my late teens where my existence depended on my contrived realities. Dan was the proverbial tall, dark, and handsome man. He was thin, even his face; not skinny really, just long and topped off with a military crew cut. By that summer of 1956, Dan had sixteen years of military service behind him and would be eligible for retirement in four more years. When we came together, in the serendipity way that two people who need each other do, I was 18 and trying to mother a one-year-old son; he had custody of two young children. He had put an eight-year marriage behind him and was still trying to forget the World War II bombing raids in Africa and Europe when I came skipping along with my own agenda.

I think for him it just made sense to bend to the swooning of a young needy girl who could mother his children. We combined our families without the blessing of a priest or magistrate and went forth into the world of pediatricians and PTAs as Mr. and Mrs. Daniel Banich and their three children, Daniel, Patricia and Gardner.

While I was choosing a house full of brand new furniture for our barracks style two bedroom rental, the salesman asked us where we were from. When he learned I was a Great Falls native, he asked me what my maiden name had been. I didn't want to admit I had been a Johnson, even though the common name was easy to hide behind, and I didn't want to talk to anyone about my Johnson past.

Dan grew up in Portland, Oregon, during the worst of the Great Depression. His father was out of the picture before Dan, the youngest of five boys, was a teenager. The boys struggled with paper routes and odd jobs to keep the family fed. The Banich boys served as altar boys in their neighborhood parish and in return the church helped their mother with food baskets. Dan's memories of those years included brushing his mother's hair that fell below her waist, having a nickel left over to go to a movie in downtown Portland, and following his older brothers on a shortcut across a railroad trestle with a train whistle blasting behind them. When he was fourteen, his mother died and the five boys were on their own. Dan believed that his mother often came to him in the form of an angel until the first time he masturbated.

So we were a Catholic family, on the surface anyway. Danny was in the second grade and it fell on me to help him prepare for his first communion. I found myself again on the outside looking into the Catholic world. Because I had married Bill in a church, and because I was baptized, that marriage was held sacred by the Church.

Danny was a sweet little boy who deserved a lot more than life handed him. Dan had taken him away from his mother when he was six, put him into an orphanage, and a year later brought him to a new home where he was told to call the young girl there "Mother." Danny was a round little fellow both physically and spiritually. Short, but proportioned nicely, he had a butch haircut like his soldier daddy. His cheeks rounded up like apples when he grinned, which he did a lot, and his eyes danced when he laughed. He wanted to be loved, and he had figured out that obedience made him loveable.

Patty looked enough like her brother to be mistaken for his twin. She had the same apple cheeks and smiling brown eyes. Patty had been barely five when her world turned upside down. She was frequently in some kind of trouble at the orphanage and in our home, too. She had long hair that needed to be curled or braided, but she didn't tolerate the grooming. After one visit with her mother, she came back with a kinky perm and a very short hair cut. I was jealous of anything her mother did, so I cut the tight curls off. Luckily, Patty looked darling in a pixie haircut. When she cut the hair off her doll, I shaved the doll's head while Patty tearfully watched.

That winter, only four months after we got together, Dan was sent to Florida on temporary assignment. I was left behind with morning sickness and three children. I'm sure the neighbors must have thought we were four children fending for ourselves. Dan taught me to drive and showed me how to use the base commissary. I conquered the mystery of the automatic washer and learned to use the dryer with the vent open after a small kitchen fire brought the fire department to our house. But I wasn't much of a mother to his children, and because I didn't want be unfair, I treated Gardner like a stepchild too. I insisted that Danny and Patty call me mom, refusing to acknowledge them unless they did. I spanked them, pulled their hair, and demanded exact obedience. Gardner wandered when he was left unattended so he had to have constant supervision. I tied him to the clothesline, and when the other two were naughty, I tied them there too. When I sent Patty to find a stick for me to spank her with, she brought back a large limb. I used it, and kept her home from school until the welts on her legs disappeared. I was nauseated, bored and lonely, and I took it out on the children.

Shirley, the children's "real" mother, as they referred to her, was a striking blond who wore spiked heels, fur coats, and huge sunglasses that made her look like a movie star. I was terribly intimidated by her, but she decided that the best way she could help her children was through me. She gave me some cooking tips, and on her weekends to have the children she sometimes took Gardner too. I grew to like her in spite of my jealous feelings. She helped me survive the long winter stuck inside with cabin fever children but when Dan came home in the spring he was mad at me for letting the children spend so much time with their mother. He reminded me that he had custody of his children because the court declared her unfit.

The 1950s were good years and I contributed to the boom of babies born during that time. The country was prosperous and even those of us who were struggling believed we would eventually achieve the American dream: a home of our own, a nice car, and maybe a Disneyland vacation. Most families attended church, and most little boys joined the Cub Scouts. Parents belonged to the PTA, and if their kids got into trouble at school, they could expect to be in trouble at home too. I washed on

Monday, ironed on Tuesday, etc. I even had underpants with the days of the week embroidered on them. We attended mass on Sunday, ate fish on Friday, and didn't use birth control.

"Topsy" 1957—1958. Five decades of harsh Montana winters have not weathered the chiseled letters in her gravestone, but the pain has blurred and my memories are faded like the old snapshot with curled edges. In the picture a young woman kneels near a mound of flowers. She wears a scarf tied tightly on her head, and clutches her fur coat close. Mt. Olivet Cemetery is treeless, and the January sky, darker than the gray horizon, meets the barren prairie in the photo. The baby's name was Jacqueline Dionne, after the famous Dionne quintuplets. The children called their baby sister Topsy, and it seemed to fit better than the formal Jacqueline. She was a welcomed bundle in our blended family and the link that made all of us related. Two boys and two girls, her birth certificate named Daniel as her father.

We moved into a huge old house with room for all of us; we even had a pantry. The bathroom had a big claw-foot bathtub that all the children could bath in at the same time. Behind the fence in our back yard were train tracks. Two-year-old Gardner figured out what time of day the trains came by, and waited on the fence to wave at the engineers who blew the whistle. Danny and Patty enrolled in public school, but continued their Catholic education at Lady of Lourdes church.

Another photo shows a chubby baby leaning against the back of a couch. A note on the back of the photo says, "Topsy could stand alone at 3 months." A drop of drool hangs on her tiny chin, and the profile shot captures a turned up nose and wisps of hair standing up in a Gerber-Baby curl. I look behind my eyes where old memories are stored, but I cannot picture my little girl of so long ago.

The big house was perfect for an old-fashioned Christmas celebration. On a trip to the woods we cut down the perfect tree, and set about decorating every room. The children put wrapping paper on the table lamps, and gleefully watched Rudolph and Frosty dance in the light when we turned them on. I made fruitcakes, popcorn balls, fudge and divinity, which Patty found and ate before the holiday, arrived. We went to school and watched Danny and Patty sing and recite the season's stories. I sewed matching black velvet jumpers for us girls to wear to midnight mass. Dan and I stayed up into those wee hours of Christmas that only parents of young children know about, putting together toys from Santa. It is a warm Christmas memory.

The winter of 1957-58 was what Montanans call open. The days were warm, and there had been only a few light showers of snow that didn't stick to the ground. The children were able to play outside and I took Gardner and Topsy on afternoon walks. By January, Topsy could sit alone and she enjoyed the stroller rides. She rarely fussed, and in fact was such a good baby that we forgot her one Sunday morning. We were all in the car on our way to church when an uneasy feeling came over me. "O my God, Dan, we forgot the baby," I screamed. When we got back to the house, she was on our bed where I had left her, just looking around.

Early in January, after the gifts were put away or broken, the man from the bank came to the house and I gave him the keys to our yellow Lincoln Continental. The car that we had had no business buying in the first place was being repossessed. Dan had lost his extra flight pay when he was transferred to the Minuteman Missile program. We were without transportation when a greater disaster struck our home.

Dan teased me when I worried about the children. He thought it was cute how I always checked on the baby while she was sleeping in her room at the top of the stairs. Sunday mornings were busy. There were pancakes to make, hairdos to fix, and clothes to pick out. That Sunday, January 19th, is written in stone and in my heart.

"It's funny the baby hasn't woke up yet," I said when I noticed it was almost nine a.m. I was actually hoping she would sleep just a little longer so that I could finish making the pancakes, but there was that feeling that all mothers know about.

"Maybe she's dead," Dan teased. He went upstairs to get her and then

I heard his steps pounding down the stairs as he screamed, "Oh, no! Oh, no! Call the doctor!"

He ran into the kitchen with the baby in his arms. I dropped the phone and tried to grab her, but Dan pulled her away from me. "It's no use!" he cried. "She's already stiff."

I screamed until his slap across my face brought me back to the kitchen and the telephone. A veil of disbelief dropped between me and what was happening. I could see the baby was not moving, and I felt her cold skin. I spoke into the phone and told the doctor that our baby looked dead.

Sirens screamed, and as the fire engines neared our house the children came running from their upstairs bedrooms. We told them to stay upstairs. Firemen rushed over to the lifeless china doll on our couch, and I watched as they put a mask on her face, and cranked the oxygen tank open. I willed her tiny fingers to move. I ran upstairs and told the children to stop laughing and playing, and to pray for their baby sister who was dying. Their faces revealed the mixed emotions of excitement and fear.

The doctor came next and made the official pronouncement of death. The priest came and baptized Topsy. He told us it might be a valid baptism because the soul didn't leave the body for three hours after death. When the undertaker arrived, he took the baby from my arms and put her body in a small metal box that looked like one of my dad's fishing tackle boxes. He handed me her blanket and told me she didn't need it; then he locked the box. That box, with my dead baby in it, sat in the middle of the living room while he wrote down the information for the obituary and burial. Then he picked up the box and left the house.

Everyone was gone. I sat in the rocker frozen. I felt like I would die too, from all the feelings I was experiencing. Dan went into our bedroom. He was there, praying and sobbing, when my sister and her husband arrived. Margaret washed my face and gave me some aspirin. She fixed lunch for the children. After they left, Dan and I gathered up the children and walked to Our Lady of Lourdes to baptize Gardner so he wouldn't die without his sacramental pass into heaven. Another family was at the church baptizing their new baby. I couldn't help staring at the live baby who fussed at the water on her head. I have often wondered what those people thought of the morose family sharing the baptismal font with them that day.

The same priest who had baptized our dead daughter tried to console us about her chances of getting to heaven versus limbo. He assured us that if she did have to reside in limbo for eternity, she would at least have eternal rest and peace, even though she would never personally know God.

Shirley took the three children home with her and kept them for a week. Friends and acquaintances stopped by with food and condolences. When Thelma and Rolph came, I begged them to stay and eat with us. I couldn't stand being left alone with my feelings. While they were there eating dinner with us I could almost believed the baby was upstairs sleeping. When they left, it was just Dan and me with pain that we couldn't share. We were frozen in our grief, unable to reach across, or through, whatever stood between us that night.

The next day the Ford dealership called and said they would give us a loaner car to drive until after the funeral. It was an Edsel, and that was the only year the model was sold. In retrospect it seems appropriate that the car they loaned us didn't live much longer than our little girl. Dan and I drove into town and met with the funeral director at a different mortuary than the one my family had gone to. We bought; I should say we charged the most expensive casket he showed us. He reminded us it was our last chance to do anything for this child. Then we bought her a white baptismal gown, and ordered flowers with ribbons that said "daughter" and "sister" on them. When we met with the priest he shamed us for wasting money on flowers that did not even make good fertilizer, and reminded us that we had three other children to care for.

When Dan had found her lying on her back with her little face tucked under the plastic crib bumpers there was blood near her nose. He believed that she had cried and struggled before she smothered, and that we didn't hear her because she was alone upstairs. The autopsy, which we had to consent to because she died unexpectedly, pointed to pneumonia. It was probably what we now know as crib death. But I thought she died because I had neglected to sterilize the tops of the milk cans that I used for her formula. I kept my secret guilt from Dan and he didn't tell me he thought she had died because we weren't married. He believed that he had been called to be a priest, and because he had refused the call, God was punishing him.

A small gathering of friends were at Topsy's short service, but only Dan and I, in the funeral car with our child's casket in the back, made the familiar trip to the cemetery. There wasn't even any snow to soften the hard land. Even the wind moaned a lonely cry that day as we drove away from the mound of dirt covered with the useless flowers.

Before Shirley brought the children back, Dan removed the crib, and I packed all of the baby's things into boxes that we took to the Salvation Army. We moved to another house and it was as though there had never been a baby.

The priest in our new parish in Black Eagle was concerned that we weren't married and that we couldn't be married in the church because of my first marriage. He said he hated to see our children lose their family but he believed we were living in a state of mortal sin. Dan's belief that Topsy had died because we weren't married seemed real to me after that so I accepted Father's directive that if we insisted on living together, we would have to live as brother and sister.

I silently said the rosary as I scrubbed the floors on my hands and knees each day, and prayed God would take our sexual desires away. He answered that prayer by sending Dan to Alaska on a temporary assignment. I was left to deny the children their right to grieve for their baby sister, and to guard our guilty secret.

Gardner regressed with his potty training and developed temper tantrums. Patty ate anything she could find in the cupboard when I wasn't looking. I raged inwardly, and outwardly I struck at the children, becoming the wicked stepmother in stories I had read to them in sweeter times. Danny started stealing and running away. He went to Shirley's, only to discover that his mother and her new husband were out of town. He crawled into their apartment through a window. A day later the police and search parties found him. They said when they went in he was sitting at the table eating crackers with peanut butter and wearing one of Art's ties. He didn't want to come home and the police asked me to try to make things easy for him until his dad returned from Alaska.

I woke up one morning to find Gardner standing at the side of my bed. On my pillow was a dead rabbit. He kept asking me why the rabbit wouldn't wake up. I don't know how the rabbit died, but after that he brought home dead chickens and once a goose. I was beside myself with grief, parenting problems, loneliness and guilt. I began having migraine headaches so severe that I pulled pieces of my hair out.

It is said that we make many acquaintances in our journey through life but only one or two friends. The gift of friendship came to me in 1958 in the long spring of my unhappiness. A family moved into the basement of the house we rented. I first met Kathy's husband, Cadet. He had not been in the United States very long and his Basque accent was heavy. It was hard for me to understand what he was saying. He had their two year old son in tow and told me that the boy, Terry, was missing his Mamma who had just given birth to twin boys. I told Cadet that Terry was welcome to come upstairs and play with my children. Terry and Gardner quickly became friends. I was in the basement laundry area when Kathy brought the twins home. We met and I held Maurice and Pierre a bit before returning to my apartment upstairs, but I was baby-starved and my arms ached to hold them. Kathy tolerated my intrusiveness and in later years confided that she didn't really realize how little time had passed since Topsy had died when we first met. She welcomed the help I was so eager to give during the early months when Pierre and Maurice needed constant care. I bought their first pair of shoes and adopted them into my heart.

Annulment papers from Bill, who was living in California, arrived. When Dan came back to Montana in July we were able to legalize our relationship. Kathy offered to take the kids while we went on a little vacation to celebrate his homecoming. For $100 Dan bought a 1949 Lincoln sedan with power windows that wouldn't stay up, and we drove to Livingston where we were married by a justice of the peace. We honeymooned in the cabins at Old Faithful in Yellowstone Park, and gave our Catholic guilt to the devil. I bought a piggy bank at the gift store at Old Faithful Lodge, and declared it was for the baby that I hoped we had started during our time in Yellowstone. When I missed my period in August, I began wearing maternity clothes.

We resumed our life as a family and normalcy came to our home once again. The children enjoyed the summer break from school in the hot Montana sunshine. They played in the sprinkler in the yard, and we took occasional trips to Mitchell Pool. We went to the State Fair where Dan and I spent our entire monthly budget in one day. We went early in the morning and stayed until after the fireworks, just as I had done with my mother. We went to the rodeo and the night show, and between those events we rode the rides and played the carnival games until each child had a large prize to carry around. The next day the kids waited in the car, while Dan and I went to Beneficial Finance to borrow grocery money.

One morning, while I was listening to soap operas on my kitchen radio I heard that a Montana woman had been among several family members killed in a tornado in Wisconsin.

"Thelma Lund was apparently killed instantly, and authorities are searching for a baby that was reported to be with her at the time the storm struck."

"Thelma? Oh, my God. My friend Thelma is dead."

She had traveled with her husband Rolph on her first ever vacation to meet his family and show them their new grandson. While Rolph's family was gathered for dinner the tornado tore across their town. Thelma's baby, little Darwin, was found alive, over 24 hours later on a piece of plywood floating in muddy water. Rolph brought Thelma's body home on the train to Irma who was crazed with the loss. Irma was emotionally out of control at Croxford's during the funeral, and collapsed at the cemetery. Her husband literally pulled her off the flower-covered casket. But then, she dried her eyes, and cared for the little boy while Rolph stayed upstairs with Thelma's things that he kept as a shrine.

I was ashamed to visit with Thelma's mother or to meet any of the people we had both known. Thelma had been everything I wasn't and I felt the others knew that. I didn't understand why she had died instead of me. Not only was I still alive, there was a new life growing inside me.

I began having vivid nightmares about tornados. I woke up screaming and drenched from sweat with those dreams for many years after Thelma's death. I was afraid to go to bed sometimes, knowing the dreams were waiting for me. My fear that a tornado would hit our family became part of my waking hours too. When the skyline darkened before a summer thunderstorm I coiled in terror. I would gather the children into the basement when a storm was approaching and play board games with them, trying to protect them from my fears. But if I couldn't find them, I hid all alone. Many, many years later I dreamed I saw the funnel cloud building on the horizon and then hanging over the skyline of downtown Great Falls. In that dream I told myself that I was dreaming, and I never had another tornado dream.

Danny, never having given up hope that he could live with his Mother again, began acting out. It seemed nothing Dan or I did made any difference in his attitude or behavior. The last straw for Dan was when Danny stole some collector coins from a neighbor. Dan, cruelly and foolishly, took him to the juvenile detention center, and then told his son—not yet ten years old—to never call him Dad again. Shirley rescued her little boy from the detention center. Later, in a multiple adoption proceeding, Shirley and Art adopted Danny and David; I adopted Patty, and Gardner became a Banich. Danny never did forgive his dad and I don't believe Patty ever got over the feeling that her mother choose Danny over her.

Patty's new birth certificate said that I had given birth to her in San Bernadino, California, when I was twelve years old. It seemed even the authorities were willing to pad my delusions. So in 1959, when I was twenty, I had a real wedding band that belonged to a real soldier, and all my children had real birth certificates.

Danette, born in March, looked very much like the sister who had died just 14 months earlier. We loved her as though she were two babies in one. She weighed less than five-and-a-half pounds and at seventeen inches long, she was a true kewpie doll. Danette had her first attack of croup at five months. Dan and I sped to the base hospital in terror with the baby whooping and gasping for breath. That was the first of so many attacks that the doctors at the base frequently admitted her for my sake more than hers.

Kathy's daughter Lisa was born in September and our friendship deepened as we shared our daughters with each other. Extra spending money was scarce so we combined ingredients from our kitchens for suppers in the winter and picnics at Giant Springs in the summer. While Kathy and I passed our morning coffee breaks over the phone, the children in both houses got into mischief and we often put our calls on hold while we spanked one or two kids. Joint spaghetti dinners often included washing the kitchen walls after eight kids slurped up the messy sauce. But those were good times.

In the spring of 1960 Dan and I made a quick trip to Astoria, Oregon where his brother, a commercial fisherman, had found a boat that the two of them hoped to purchase. The plan was to go into partnership when Dan retired in 1964.

While we were in Oregon, the children and I went to the Tongue Point Navy Station to see a presidential candidate who was stopping there that day. I would be voting for the first time, and I planned on voting for the dashing young John F. Kennedy. I thought his wife, Jacqueline, was so sophisticated, and I wanted to see little children living in the White House. The helicopter was late, and although we did grow tired of waiting, it turned out to be a historical day for the Banich family. John F. Kennedy shook our hands and patted Danette on the head.

Soon after Danette's second birthday, another little boy joined our family. On his second day of life the doctor said, "Your baby has a defective heart, but he seems healthy otherwise." I was not able to take a deep breath for over a year. When I took the pale little baby home, I tried not to let him cry because his lips and his fingernails turned blue when he did. We made monthly trips to the doctor for EKGs but Francis thrived and by his second year the murmur had disappeared. Kathy bonded with Francis in a special way. She was tired of babies but she said there was something special about him. Kathy had what could be called an ample bosom and he cupped around her softness when she held him and was quiet and contented.

I read every magazine and newspaper I could find with anything about Jackie Kennedy, and her children. I copied her style. I cut Danette's hair like Caroline's, and Francis had the famous John-John bowl hair cut. My little ones both wore white high-top shoes, and little coats I made from material salvaged from Salvation Army donations. They had matching Easter outfits. Dan and I doted on those two toddlers more than we should have. Meanwhile, Gardner was growing into a schoolboy with a shock of bright red hair and freckles everywhere.

That summer Kathy insisted that I made amends with my estranged dad. We went to skid row together and as I walked through the bars and taverns in search of the man I had adored as a child my heart softened. He was living in a room over the Club Cigar Store. He had a large abdominal hernia that made him look pregnant and his pants were unzipped, tied together with a string and he let his shirt hang over the gap. The ring of hair circling his head had turned gray, but other than that he was still Daddy. He still tied fishing flies. He sold the flies and dealt cards now and then to get by. He seemed grateful that I had come to visit him, and promised to come and meet my family when could buy decent clothes. He kept that promise and when the children gathered around their newfound grandpa it was good thing.

The United States and Russia were posturing in the seas around Cuba in the fall of 1961, and because we lived on the military base, we were very much aware of the imminent danger. The base held practice evacuations, and we had to keep food and water in a makeshift bomb shelter in the basement. At school the children practiced crawling under their desks if the sirens went off. I lived on the edge of terror that month, and worried that our children might not be reunited with us if we evacuated to an outlying area while they were in school. Dan was working underground in the Minuteman Missile Silos. These missiles, deep in the ground in sites throughout central Montana, were equipped with warheads. Given the command, the huge concrete covers would open and the missiles would lift off in search of programmed targets. The United States also had airplanes in the air loaded with nuclear weapons. Dan, an informed military person, was rightfully worried, and announced to me that when, and if the current crisis ended, he wanted the children and me to move to Oregon. He said I could be looking for a home in Astoria while he finished his last year before retirement.

President Kennedy and his brother, Robert, the Attorney General, forced the Russians streaming towards Cuba to turn around, averting what could have been the start of World War III.

While Dan and I watched the evening news reports and held our breath in fear, my Dad was losing his own battle. A nurse at the County Hospital called to tell me that my Dad had been admitted and that he was dying of lung cancer. I took cigarettes, unfiltered Lucky Strikes, and I listened to his dream to build a small cabin on Sheep creek where he could catch fish and fry them up for breakfast every morning.

The phone rang one day in October, two years before Daddy's Social Security checks would have begun; my father had expired that morning. I made the familiar trip to Croxford's, chose the casket, and made the necessary arrangements. The funeral director, probably Dennis, who had gone to school with me, didn't urge me to buy the best. Daddy had died penniless in the County Hospital and I, his only relative, was living from paycheck to paycheck. The welfare package was predetermined: a simple but respectable casket, the service room, and funeral cars for the trip to Highland Cemetery's paupers' section.

The services were short with recorded music behind the velvet drapes and a minister, who offered his services free, eulogized a man he had never met. Goldie came with her new boy, my sister and a few of Daddy's cronies from downtown barely filled the large room. Aunt

Eula and Uncle Hobart met me at the cemetery with many hugs and memories. I left not only my dad at Highland Cemetery, but also my heritage. It would be the last time I would see anyone from my Johnson past.

I moved to Oregon the next spring. We visited with my sister a couple of days before we left and she was sad to see that I was pregnant again.

"Carol," she chided, "those cute babies turn into children you know."

I said I would write to her. Dan put a piece of plywood across the back seat of our car so the children could play and sleep back there on the drive to Oregon. Patty, who had to fold her long legs under her, was feeling bad about leaving her mother behind and I felt awful about moving away from my friends. We stayed overnight at Cadet and Kathy's so we could leave early the next morning but there were many false starts as tears and hugs were exchanged. I cried all the way across Montana on that Mother's Day in 1963.

We found a two-bedroom apartment in the country not far from the Columbia River. The complex was converted military barracks housing and several young families were living there. Dan made sure our car was running well, and then he took the bus back to Montana. He assured me he would be back when the baby came in July. I felt desperately alone.

CHAPTER 12—ASTORIA

I wondered, during my first wet spring in Oregon, if Lewis and Clark had arrived in Astoria as I had, exhausted from the trials and tribulations that brought them there; incredibly lonesome for home, yet overwhelmed by the pristine beauty of the Columbia River country.

Astoria sits on forested hills surrounded by rivers and bays. Huge spruce and cedar trees glisten with the moisture of heavy fog, which either thins enough for rays of sun to play among the trees, or thickens to sift a steady mist onto ferns and moss-covered ground below. The Columbia River, a gathering of waters from the slopes of the Continental Divide, flows deep and wide with purpose and determination toward the Pacific Ocean. There, the river struggles to pass through the crashing waves of the bar to complete its westward journey. Having reached their nirvana, the waters evaporate and cumulous gatherings either dip low and weep over the coastal range, or rage their way back to the mountains on fierce winds.

Astoria and the surrounding villages are fishing communities. It seemed like a foreign country, with strange words and sounds. Fishing boats bobbed at the piers, or were unloading their catch at the fish canneries. Ferry boats sounded their warnings as they maneuvered to unload cars from the Washington side of the river. An orchestra of harbor noises, shrouded by fog, played as the vessels wound their way through buoys and jetties, sounding their horns for safe passages.

I looked through homesick tears at soggy brown leaves that refused to let go of their place on trees that were pushing them away with new growth. Mrs. Banich, as the grocer called me when I brought the four children in to shop, was nearly twenty-five-years old. I look at a photo of me and the children and I see a young woman who, despite her pregnancy, is slim and quite pretty. My curly auburn hair is cropped short and capped around my high forehead in a way that softens the freckles that haven't faded yet. I wear a small pill hat with a half-veil in preparation for church that day. Patty, thick brown hair falling across her face, bends to tend to Danette, enjoying her role as mother's helper. She is entering her teens with deep brown eyes and feather-thick lashes above high cheek bones that hinted, even then, of the beautiful woman she would become. Danette, the family princess, poses pretty in a French- blue velvet dress; little Francis, peeking shyly through his blond circle of bangs wears a matching Eton suit. They are the darlings, the faux Kennedy children. Gardner, a splatter of rust colored freckles competing with his burnt orange crew cut, looks at the photographer through black horn-rimmed glasses. My firstborn is almost nine, and although I ask him to be in charge of Francis I know I can't depend on him. He is easily distracted, and rushes in where any angel would fear to tread.

The children settled into our new life with the resiliency of youth. Gardner soon had a box of water snakes on the back porch that I inventoried each night to make sure none were in his bed. Danette, enrolled in a dance class, practiced her tap lesson, "One to three, look at me, I can tap my toe," followed by three taps with the metal toed shoes. Patty, applauded the first dozen or so successful taps, and then returned to her latest baking project. Patty kept her little brothers and sister supplied with cookies and cakes, though it threatened my small grocery budget. Francis played with his cars in whatever quiet corner he could find in our crowded apartment.

Although I joined the neighbors in their coffee klatches, melancholy plagued me. I missed my friend Kathy. We spoke to each other by phone a few times but the calls grew further apart as distance severed our emotional ties. I waited impatiently for the baby to be born so that Dan would come. I missed his help with the children, and I missed the evening cup of coffee we shared after tucking the kids into bed. Dan was a good father, doing without his cigarettes if we needed spending money before the next payday. He supported me in the care and training of the children, but I wondered if he welcomed the frequent temporary assignments that took him across the world for weeks at a time.

The familiar labor pains began their slow crescendo on July 26, I deposited the children with a neighbor, called Dan, and drove to the hospital. Stephen Marcus came easily into the world even though, at almost eight pounds, he was my biggest baby. Dan arrived in time to take us home and when he pulled up to the hospital with the four older children, the Sister who wheeled me out to the car told me that if I had two more children, I would earn a star in my Heavenly crown.

Dan stayed in Oregon until the middle of August. Although I knew he would be back for Christmas, I felt lonely before he even boarded the bus. The smaller children soon figured out that when I was nursing the new baby they could get into mischief. I was unable to do anything but yell at them and after they wandered into the street one day, I decided Stephen would have to be a bottle baby. He probably didn't suffer any lasting damage from propped bottle feedings, but I think that was when my unstoppable tears began. I cried into the pillow at night, and in the morning tears ran into my ears as I summoned the energy to get up to face another day. A neighbor with a little boy Francis's age noticed the changes in my children's appearance and when they played on the porch in the rain all afternoon one day she knocked on my door to ask if I was all right. She said she had noticed that the children had been outside for a long time and wondered if I was ill. I told her I was tired and that I just couldn't quit crying ever since the last baby was born. She made a pot of coffee and offered me one of her cigarettes .She sat there without saying much and just let me cry. When I ended what I called my pity-pot, she said with a sigh, "God, girl, I would cry all the time too if I had as many kids as you do and no man around to help. Where the hell is your husband anyway?"

When I explained our plans she blurted out, "What an asshole thing for him to do."

I tried to tell her that I had been part of the plan that brought me to Oregon early, but she lit another cigarette and dropped the subject.

After that, my new friend and I drank a lot of coffee and smoked a lot of cigarettes together, and I didn't cry as much. In October as the date that Dan I celebrated our anniversary neared, she began teasing me about going out dancing and drinking to celebrate without "the asshole." The anniversary fell on a Friday night, and that cinched it for her. On Fridays there was always a live band and we were going dancing! We hired Patty to watch all the kids, and I went out on the town with my friend and her husband. I hadn't danced since I lived in Sweet Grass, but I got my rhythm back with the beat of the drums and only one drink. When the young grocer leaned away from his dance partner and said "Hello, Mrs. Banich," I laughed and told him it was my wedding anniversary. That prompted him to ask the band to play the "Anniversary Waltz," and we danced together while I explained where Mr. Banich was. It was fun and although we went home early, I didn't have to be coaxed to go again the next Friday.

Patty enjoyed having spending money, and at first I never left her with the children until they were all in bed. My circle of party friends grew. I was going out at least two nights every week, and one drink no longer was enough.

I sobered up with the rest of our nation that fateful afternoon of November 22 in 1963. I was watching soap operas and I gasped in disbelief when the program was interrupted with the news that President Kennedy had been shot. After I ran around the complex knocking on doors to tell everyone who had missed the news flash, I took my place, with the entire country, in front of the television set and watched in numbed disbelief as the events unfolded. I cried as I watched my heroine, Jacqueline Kennedy, in her bloody pink clothes look out at the nation through lifeless eyes. Patty and Gardner, who had been excused from school, sat with me. We watched the horse-drawn hearse, followed by Jackie veiled in black, make its way down the streets of our nation's Capitol. I watched with a mother's heart as John-John said goodbye to his daddy with a chubby hand salute. Camelot was gone and the demise of the Banich family was not far behind.

Dan came for Christmas, and for a week all was right with the world, but after Christmas the winter rains came. The nearby hills were smothered in dense fog, and the sky dripped continuously. I danced and drank at the nightclub, and not just on Fridays. One night I accepted a ride home from the guitar player. Patty was awake and saw me necking with him in the car. When I came into the house, she ran out of the bedroom, wild eyed and sobbing, "I saw you! I saw you, Mom!"

I denied what she had seen and calmed her down with hugs and reassurances. Our mutual denial formed an everlasting wedge between us.

Riddled with guilt and shame, I accepted an invitation to attend a prayer service at an evangelical church in town. When the altar call began with the usual, Just as I Am, I went forward and sobbed at the railing while strangers prayed for me to give my heart to Jesus Christ. One of those praying for me was a young pastor whom I gave my heart to instead of Jesus.

The Nazarene Church in Astoria was his first pastoral assignment. He was eager to save our little family; not only from Catholicism, but also from Astoria's nightlife. He looked like John Ritter, the minister in The Waltons. He was handsome in a wholesome boyish way and as naïve as he appeared. I soon was singing in the choir, and helping to paint a day care center, and doing as much volunteer work as I could, and as little mothering as possible. When the pastor whispered to me from the back row during choir practice that he could still smell cigarette smoke on me, I thrilled at the attention. When my washing machine broke down and my old car stopped running, he came to the housing complex and helped me load soggy diapers and mounds of laundry into his car and took me to the laundromat. When I manipulated the circumstances so he would know I was in the bar drinking, he came and with an arm around my shoulders he took me home to my children. He knelt with me in my home and prayed for me.

I was swinging wider and wider with my emotions. I wanted to be in both worlds at the same time. My first choice would have been the church, but my new crush was married and had children. My attraction to him was enormous, but not sexual. I just wanted to be held by him forever. In my mind, he was goodness personified, and I craved the unconditional love he professed to offer me. I faked a suicide attempt when I knew he was coming over to pick me up for some function. He found me on the couch, incoherent, with aspirins scattered on the floor. Sobering me up with coffee and making me walk was very effective, because I had nothing in my system expect deceit. His wife came and took my children to the parsonage, and after many prayers and promises from me he went home to his family. I had promised him I would see a mental health counselor.

With guilt as my constant companion, I may have been closer to suicide than I realized. There were times I drove my car at speeds over 110 miles an hour, wrestling with the desire to turn the wheel sharply into the hell where I belonged. I began going to the local mental health center once a week. I talked about fears and concerns, but not mine. I kept trying to gain control of my deteriorating family. Patty was confused as I demanded prayers but they were not the prayers she had learned in Catechism classes. Forced into too many responsibilities, she was beginning to express her resentment openly. Gardner happily ran wild. One bit of humor, out of this family tragedy, is still shared at family gatherings. Gardner raided the neighbor's goldfish pond before I came home one night, probably drunk. I didn't see pink elephants, but goldfish, one in each one of my pots and pans scattered across the kitchen floor.

Stephen was and still is our mellow fellow, so he thrived in spite of the neglect during his first few months. Some days I would promise myself I was going to make a turn for the good. I would begin by arranging all of the toddler's toys in order, by color or size, on their shelves, or I would take the clothes out of the closets and put them back in colored categories. As my obsessive work was undone by the children's normal activities, my anxiety increased and escaped in the form of rage. One morning I discovered the septic tank had backed up outside and pink toilet-paper wads that looked like wet cotton candy were strewn about the soggy yard. When the pastor arrived to take me to my mental health appointment it was too late in many ways. I was sitting in the middle of that mess sobbing, picking at the slimy mess and wanting to die.

The therapist at the mental health center tried to convince me to continue with outpatient support, but I begged to enter the state hospital in Salem for a thirty day trial. People in the church agreed to keep my children. I packed a box for each child; favorite blankets and rattles for baby Stephen, toy cars and bibbed overalls for Francis and favorite dresses for Danette who hated pants. Patty packed her own things, everything she owned went into several boxes. She announced she would never live with me again. Gardner refused to pack anything, demanding to know where he was going and why. I told him to go with the lady who was waiting, and stop asking questions. I watched from the kitchen window as that stranger walked down the street with my baby in her arms, Francis holding her hand and Gardner trudging behind her with frequent looks back at our house. The pain I felt that day was welcomed. I savored the bittersweet scene as a karmic reward for all that I wasn't. Gardner couldn't see my tears that day, but he felt them for the rest of his life.

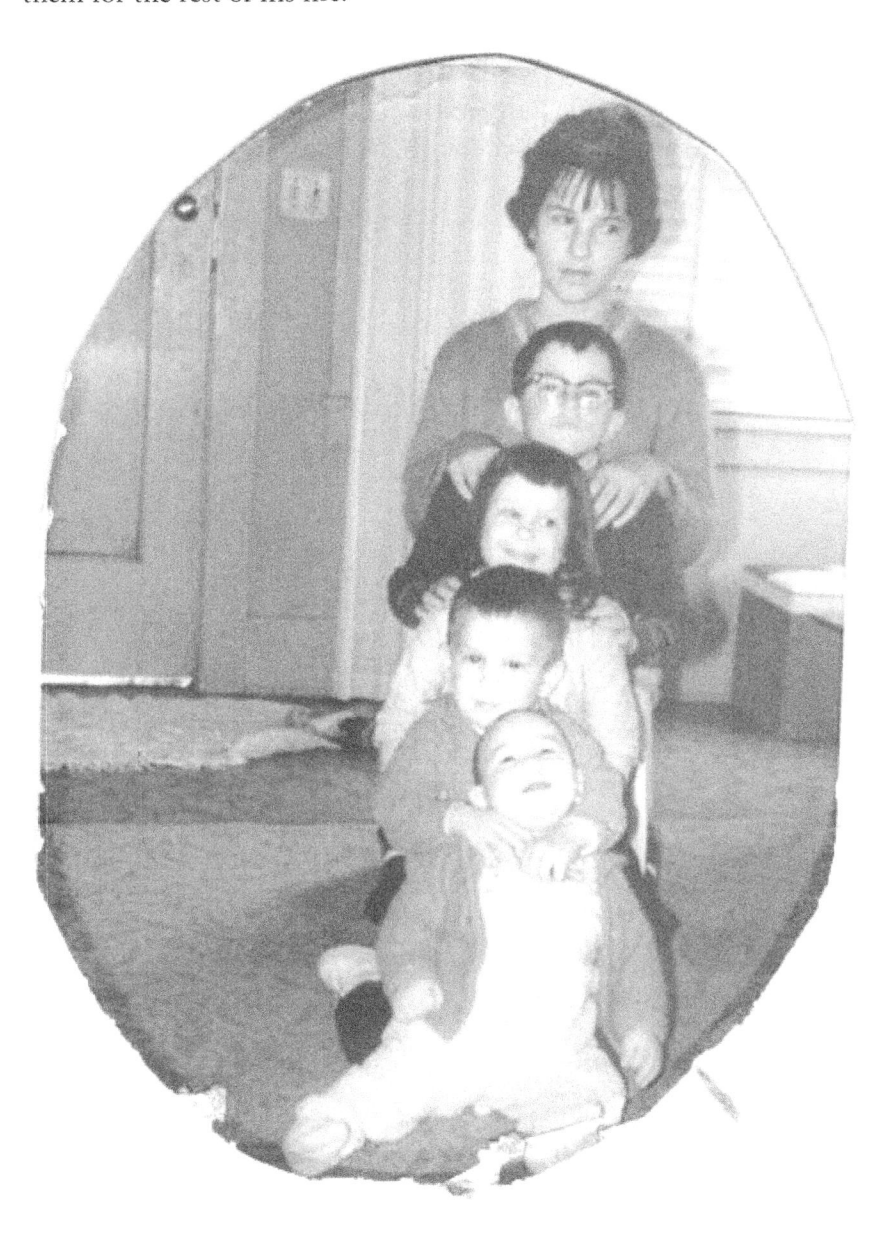

The girls settled with people they knew. Patty was old enough to understand that I wasn't well, but Danette, my thumb sucking, tender, well-behaved little darling, curled up into herself and is still there in that safe place. A picture of the five children reveals their emotions. Patty looks away, and her limp hands on Gardner's shoulders show her helpless resignation. Gardner sets his face in stone, defying his feelings. The three little cuties happily smile for the camera, not realizing this family will be frozen in time forever.

CHAPTER 13—THE CUCKOO LANDS

The Cuckoo's Nest was filmed on the grounds and in the buildings of The Oregon State Hospital. That was my destination and I feared my destiny. My pastor pushed the buzzer near the front door. We saw a man dressed in white remove a large ring of keys from his belt. He unlocked the door and took my suitcase. We followed him into the nurse's station. I felt like I was floating near the ceiling and watching the admitting process going on below me. I signed a voluntary commitment form agreeing to stay thirty days. The attendant listed of all of my things and put them into a plastic basket. He told me I'd get everything back as soon as it was marked with my name. I wanted to go out to eat supper with the pastor before he went back to Astoria, but the attendant said it wasn't a good idea.

Hospital patients, both curious and curious looking, leaned over the top stair railing as I was escorted to the second floor. I followed the uniformed matron through a room and most of the patients, deep in their own insanity, didn't even look up. The matron, a middle-aged woman who chewed her bottom lip between words, showed me the communal showers and the toilet stalls with half doors. I followed her till she stopped near the end of a hall where she showed me the room I would be sharing with two other women. Three iron beds with pastel coverlets had nearby nightstands. The matron tried to introduce me to a woman on one beds.

"Mabel, Mabel. Hey, Mabel stop that and listen to me," she said interrupting the woman's obvious masturbation maneuvers.

"This is your new roommate. Her name is Carol. You make sure Carol knows when to go to supper, and show her where the dining room is."

Mabel stared at the matron. Her skin sagged around her open mouth, and she appeared half-drugged as she tipped her head back to see beneath droopy eyelids.

"She'll show you." the matron reassured me and left the room.

Mabel went back to her activities and I lay down on the bed and cried into the pillow until she said: "Come on. It's dinner time."

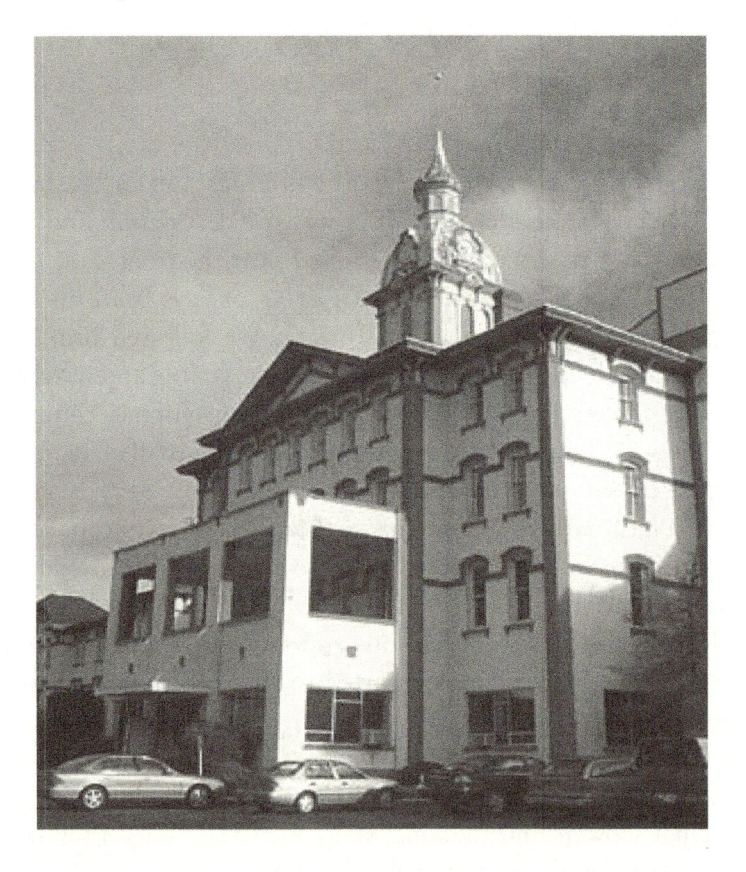

The large dining room with windows around three sides had about twenty-five round tables with colored tablecloths and cloth napkins set up for family-style meals. I took my place in the line outside and trembled with terror when a thin mute man named Wilbur pushed me out of the way. When I got back in line, I was behind a woman who took about three steps forward, stopped, mumbled to herself, then shook her head and retreated back three steps. She didn't seem to mind when I cut ahead of her. She was still trying to get to the dining room when the rest of us were seated. An attendant took her arm and forced her to a table, where she performed the same dance with her fork. That gray-haired lady, who constantly ironed her cotton housedress with hands that were bloody from constant hand washing, had been a schoolteacher before her breakdown.

Each building at the hospital was named for the county from which its patients were admitted. The Clatsop unit, where I would live, housed both men and women of all ages and diagnoses. Many were people who had coped with multiple setbacks and losses, but, like me I suppose, caved in under the proverbial last straw. Some had suffered head injuries, like the nine-year-old boy hurt in a bicycle accident who would never leave the hospital. Others were nonfunctioning either because of the intensity of their illness, or because of lobotomies or castrations. I learned not to sit at a table with anyone who drooled, picked their nose and ate it, or had feces on their fingernails.

When I arrived the hospital looked much like it did when the movie was made in 1975. The 148-acre campus sits within the city limits of Salem, Oregon and the main building, called "J," a 500,000 square-foot two-story building, borders Center Street. In the past, people driving by the hospital at night were able to look through windows covered by harlequin-shaped security bars, at men shuffling around the day room holding up cotton pants issued to them without the forbidden drawstrings. The second story of the building was where Ward 38, which housed the criminally insane, was located. Outside, behind Ward 38 was a basketball court with rolled barbed wire at the top of the fenced area. Down the alley from that exercise area there was a canteen, a gathering place for patients who had a little spending money and ground privileges. Patients on their way to the canteen shouted obscenities and other rude comments at men in the secured playground. Winter guests, those alcoholics and homeless individuals who signed in each fall when the temperatures began to drop; whiled away the winter in the canteen, drinking coffee, smoking and swapping stories. On Saturday, the hospital showed a movie there, and for some patients that was their date night, a chance to hold hands or steal a kiss in the dark. Those who wanted to do more than hold hands went underground for "tunnel therapy."

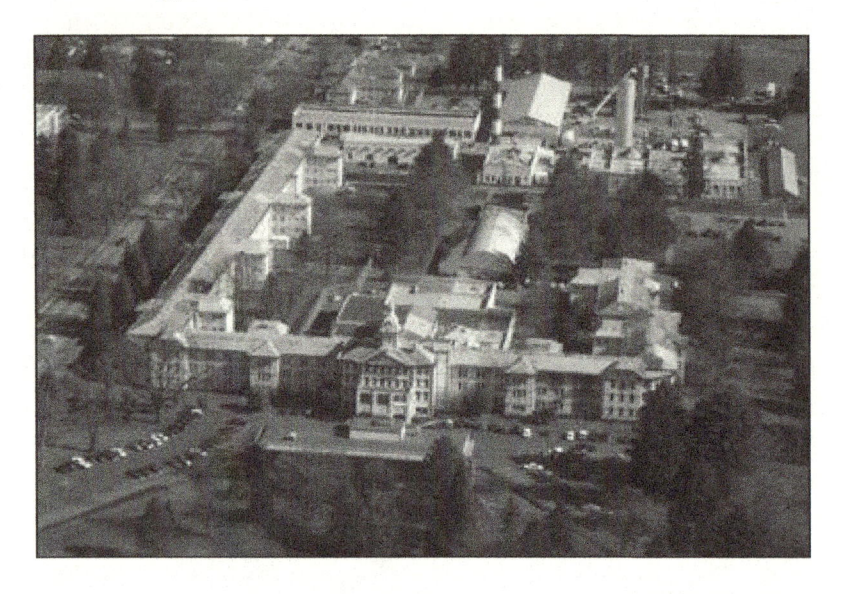

Under the hospital's buildings, deep in the ground, are three miles of tunnels that provided movement from building to building. Patients in shackles who were moved from one building to another for appointments or activities; traveled via those tunnels to protect the sensitive general public. The tunnels were also used for transporting supplies and as a dry passage for employees and medical personnel during inclement weather. There were remnants of the hospital's hideous past in those tunnels. With no psychotropic drugs to sedate them, the insane were chained or kept in wire cages. I saw rusty pieces of chains dangling from metal rings bolted into rotting posts, and I imaged half-naked, wild-haired, men and women held in those dank tunnels until their manic phase gave way to depression or they were too exhausted to cry out. Scratches and scrapes on the calcimined walls screamed out from another time.

Some of the people I met during my time at Oregon State Hospital included a man who had worked in the main kitchen back in 1942. He accidentally, perhaps, put cockroach poisoning into the scrambled eggs. Forty-four of the 467 patients and staff sickened from the contaminated eggs died. He was considered a mass murderer by his fellow patients, and treated as a pariah until his death in 1982.

An older man who monitored the men's linen closet also worked in the shops where he washed and detailed the hospital vehicles, including the fire engine that he drove to Noble's Tavern one summer afternoon. The hospital security guys found him sitting at the bar enjoying a cool beer. He was a tiny man who always wore a blue chambray shirt and denim bib overalls. He kept his white hair and mustache trimmed, and he spoke softly. He had been at the hospital for over thirty years. On the wall in the linen room, he kept a picture of his graduating class where he was standing next to his famous classmate, Albert Einstein.

Johnny, an obese boyish-man, appeared to be retarded. He would put his big hands around someone's neck, and when that person complained Johnny giggled as he ran away. As a teenager he had gone hiking with two girls, and was the only one who came out of the woods that day. The girls were found dead from strangulation.

I made friends with a woman in her early twenties who was found running up and down the freeway in Portland with nothing on. She insisted she did that to win a bet she made with her hippie friends that she could fake mental illness. We had the same psychiatrist, a young doctor working at his first job. He was easily flustered and we tormented him as much as we could. He decided to give my friend Sodium Pentothal, which is also called truth serum, because her story about faking was quite convincing. I sat in the exam room during the administration of the drug because my new friend asked for me to be there. I was stunned when she began to cry and told a story about jumping from a car because her boyfriend had promised to take her to hell and he turned the wrong direction. Her torturous delusional story went on and on. After that the doctor scheduled her for ECT, electric shock therapy. ECT was believed to separate the patient from the part of the brain that held the insane thoughts. During the weeks of treatment, my talented friend forgot how to play the piano, lost control of her bladder and appeared much worse. I mourned the loss of my friend, and I hated the young man who had the authority to do this to her. Like the sister of an abused sibling, I feared the man who could do the same damage to me. But my friend slowly regained her intellect and talents, and when she left the hospital, she had become a lovely young lady none of us had known before. I was impressed with her recovery but I didn't want ECT to be included in my therapy. Actually, I was never put on any medications. I attended group sessions and had individual sessions with the psychiatrist. I didn't think I was crazy, yet I felt fragile, and I was afraid to leave the hospital. When it came time to sign the next commitment paper, I had to agree to stay 90 days. The doctor said I needed time out, a recess from my life. He explained that the word asylum meant a safe place.

For the first time in my young adulthood I had time for me, time to take a bath uninterrupted—albeit in a bathroom without a door —and time to enjoy a meal prepared by someone else. Sometimes I ached to hold my babies, and I couldn't bear to think I might never be with them again. I threw their photographs down the hall one time and broke the glass in the frames. When I lost control like that, I was rewarded with an injection that put me to sleep. I had migraine headaches for which I received pain-killing injections that gave me psychedelic nightmares.

Dan called the hospital and he was furious. He accused me of being hysterical to get attention. He said didn't believe in psychiatry. He told me I should have gone to the priest in Astoria. My protestant pastor had called Dan, foolishly thinking Dan would understand why I had broke down, but Dan was enraged. Not only about his children being placed in Pentecostal homes, but also that I had turned to another man for help. In March, just weeks before Dan would retire from the Air Force, I received divorce papers. They had been drawn up in Conrad, Montana. The children were not named in those papers and although the papers were served to me at the mental hospital, that didn't seem to be a problem with that court. To keep me from getting part of Dan's military pension, the divorce had to take place before his retirement date. I signed the papers.

My sister called and angrily pointed out that I didn't have to be in the hospital just because I wanted a divorce and that I should get the hell out of there and grow up.

Shirley went to court in Astoria, and gained custody of Patty. She tried to convince the courts to let her take Danette back to Spokane with her too, but the welfare system wouldn't let her do that. Shirley brought all of the children to the hospital to visit me. Danny sat across the table in the visiting room pretending he wasn't there, and Patty—who was happy to get out of the foster home she was in—sobbed for me and her brothers and sister. Gardner and Danette kept asking me when I was going to come home. Francis clung to me, refusing to give up his spot in my lap to baby Stephen who innocently played at my feet. After Patty moved, Danette went to live in the same foster home as her brothers. She moved seven more times before our nightmare ended in 1968.

I wandered aimlessly through the day rooms, and sat through group sessions that seemed a waste of time. Group therapy consisted of sitting with a psychiatric aide who tried to lead a therapeutic conversation with one or two verbal patients and several head-bobbing droolers. When some student nurses sat in on our group one of them asked me why I spoke about my children without using their names. She asked me to say their names so I rattled off the seven names like a school child might recite the ABCs. The student kept probing me to share my feelings. I picked up a glass ashtray, and threw it across the room; I was given extra time with my doctor for that outburst and in that session, he challenged me to come up with one word that described love. I didn't understand his request, and even when he answered for me, I didn't fully understand how love and caring could be the same.

Johnny wasn't the only patient on our unit who had killed someone. Sometimes after years on the criminally insane unit, patients improved enough to move to an open unit. George Holly had been sentenced to the criminally insane unit in 1961. He was moved to the Clatsop unit late in 1963. George was a large man who walked softly in his bulky 6 foot, 5-inch frame. In any other setting he could easily have been mistaken for a professional. His broad shoulders filled out the institutional shirts, and he tucked the shirt-tails in, perhaps to draw attention to his physique. He had gray hair that had receded into a horseshoe-shape and sideburns grew past his ears. I thought he was very good-looking. A tight-mouth smile belied the twinkle in his eyes. I watched him whenever we were in the same room, trying to be careful so he wouldn't catch me staring. We spoke to each other now and then, but I kept my curiosity to myself until one day when we were alone in the kitchen.

"Could I ask you something?" I said, trying to sound nonchalant.

He was reaching into the fridge; I saw the muscles on his jaw tighten, but I went on, "Is it true that you killed a man?"

He took a glass out of the cupboard, poured some milk into it, and put the carton back into the refrigerator. Then he turned, looked directly at me and said; "Sure, a lot of people kill other people everyday on the highway or some other way. So what's the big deal if I killed someone?" he challenged.

"I, I guess you're right," I stammered. Although we continued to talk to each other after that, neither of us brought the tender subject up again for a long time.

My sense of absolute security within my asylum was ripped out from under me when I was slapped with a dose of reality by my psychiatrist. I had walked away from the hospital grounds with another patient, but when no one came after us with sirens and handcuffs, we walked back to the hospital. Another time I threw a full-blown temper tantrum in the dining room—throwing dishes at the windows and screaming out of control—until four male attendants carried me to the quiet room and strapped me to a bare mattress with leather restraints. It is hard to explain why it felt good to be restrained, but it did. It was almost sensual. The next morning, my psychiatrist came to the room and unlocked the restraints. I couldn't believe it when he said I would either have to straighten up and take advantage of my time in therapy, or I would have to leave the hospital. Huh! I couldn't believe what he said. How could he kick me out? I signed a contract for 90 days, and he knew I didn't have anywhere to go. I started to protest, but he stopped me. He told me I had jeopardized the safety of the patient I had taken off campus, and I wasn't making any effort to return to my children who were being cared for by the state while I played patient.

"It's time for you to grow up," he said before he walked out of the room.

I made an appointment with the social worker and we talked about my future. I didn't have any plans, but I knew I was supposed to, so I agreed to take a battery of vocational tests. My IQ was high, and other tests indicated that I could pursue almost any course of studies that I wanted to. I enrolled in a GED class and I spent more and more time with George. He was a patient tutor. My social worker suggested I consider going to a school in Klamath Falls where I could take a two-year class to be certified as a medical lab tech. Meanwhile, I grew more and more attracted to George and I wanted to know what had happened before he came to the hospital. I didn't want ask him about it. I narrowed my search to the summer of 1961 and found the July 16 headlines in the Oregon Statesman.

"Druggist Killer Suspect Jailed."

A druggist in Cannon Beach had been bludgeoned to death with a fifteen inch iron timber bolt.

"Oregon State Police arrested Holly who they found incoherent and apparently suffering from shock and exposure in a cabin he had broken into about a mile from Cannon Beach."

They found his abandoned car and were able to identify him with documents found in the car.

"Doctors said the 250 pound ex-Air Force man and former psychiatric patient was talking as though he was still in Korea."

I didn't tell George I about my search at the library, but as our friendship grew he told me more about what he "remembered." He told me he had been drinking with a man that night and when the man said to George, "There is more to this than meets the eye, Horatio," George realized he knew that George had figured out Einstein's theory of relativity. George said no one was supposed to know that he had that knowledge, and there was nothing to do but kill the man. I wasn't sure what I wanted to believe. On the one hand, I wanted to believe that George was clever enough to fake his mental illness to get out of an accidental murder that he committed during a drunken brawl. But, on the other hand, I had to admit he had a past psychiatric history. Yet maybe he was falling back on that history to support his defense—innocent by reason of insanity—his only chance to have the charges dropped. His attorney would take his insanity plea back to the courts in Astoria once the state hospital determined he was mentally competent to stand trial.

George's parents stood by him, never giving a hint of what they believed about the murder. They hired a high-profile attorney in Portland. George explained to me that he was given a psychiatric disability from the Air Force because of a suicide attempt. While he was stationed in Hawaii, he observed one of the hydrogen bomb tests at Eniwetok. He said he couldn't explain the effect that had on him. He was unable to shake his belief in an impending doomsday, and he said that painful anxiety was the reason he walked into the surf in a suicide attempt.

After going through insulin shock therapy, he was discharged from the Air Force and because he was ashamed to face his parents, he stayed lost in the hills and canyons of Northern California. Then he drifted up the coastline and landed in Cannon Beach.

George was a model patient. He attended group, he charmed the psychiatrist and nurses, and he cheeked his pills successfully. He put together a small woodworking shop on the unit, and made birdhouses and other craft items that he sold in the hospital gift shop. He had a radio in the shop, and except for some of the droolers who shuffled through the shop in their cotton slippers, no one bothered him. It was there that we fell in love. I decided not to travel to southern Oregon to go to school because I wanted to be near the hospital until he was freed.

As soon as I passed the GED, I enrolled in a business college in Salem where I where I took secretarial classes. I learned to type and to take shorthand, but I never really picked up any speed in those skills. I did well with bookkeeping and correspondence classes, and I took part time classes at a charm school. Because I wasn't a resident of Oregon when I entered the hospital, I couldn't get funding to move into my own apartment or the YWCA. So I stayed on at the hospital while I attended school; I had to check in before eight each evening.

I had a kidney infection when I was carrying Stephen and I was still having periodic infections. I was sent to the University of Oregon's Medical School in Portland and had many tests. Cobalt was injected into my veins and the radioactive material was tracked with a Geiger counter. A tube threaded through my femoral artery and up into my heart allowed dye injected into my arteries to be seen on a screen and the medical team came to the conclusion that I was born with only one kidney.

The doctors cautioned me not to risk another pregnancy. My psychiatrist asked me if I would consider having my tubes tied. I was beginning to fantasize a future with George who made no secret about his dislike for children so I gave in and agreed to be sterilized.

Dr. Dean Brooks, the same hospital superintendent who portrayed himself in the movie, sat in the front seat of the state car with the security guard who drove us to Portland. Dr. Brooks presented me to the members of the Oregon State Board of Eugenics. The members were superintendents of Oregon institutions. When we arrived in the conference room, Dr. Brooks took his seat on the other side of a long table. I sat alone on the other side. The board members, all older men, asked me if I knew what it meant to be sterilized. They asked me lots of other questions about my children, my husband, and my plans for the future and my health. They approved the hospital's request for my sterilization, and I signed the papers.

Thirty-eight years later Oregon's Governor, John Kizhaber, scheduled a special ceremony on December 2, 2002, to acknowledge the hundreds of Oregonians who were sterilized by the state. Until 1967, sterilization had often been used as a condition of release from state institutions. While my situation fell short of a forced sterilization, I was coerced to cooperate. The sterilization records of the Board of Eugenics and its successor, the Board of Social Protection, were shredded to erase proof of one of the state's most troubling chapters. The history of what happened depends on the memory of those of us who were there. Former members of the Board of Eugenics, chiefly the superintendents of state institutions who met quarterly, have hazy or incomplete recollections. Dr. Brooks, explaining that it was forty years ago, said he could only remember a handful of people being sterilized. I can only remember one person for sure, but I remember it well.

Dan brought Gardner to visit me in the spring of 1965, but I was in town attending class. George told the charge nurse that I didn't want to see Dan. I wonder if Dan and I might have reconstructed our family had I been there that day.

George dominated me with hypnosis, I think. I never felt like I was hypnotized, but I've read that others who have been hypnotized didn't think they really were. During one of those sessions in the corner of his woodshop, he talked me back to my childhood. He told me I was on an island made of clouds where there was an emerald pool. He baptized me and told me I would be pure and brand new when I woke up.

I finished business school, and was immediately hired by the state hospital to work as a secretary for the volunteer service department. I moved into the nurse's quarters, and George brazenly carried some furniture across the campus and up the stairs to my room, looking very much like he knew what he was doing. We made love all afternoon, consummating our year-long relationship. He gave me a large diamond ring that he said his mother picked out for me, and we became a couple with an uncertain future. I didn't know the ring was fake but I think some of the people I showed it to did.

George returned to court in Astoria, and was found not guilty by reason of insanity. He was sentenced to remain in the hospital until doctors determined he was safe to be in the community. We were married in the spring of 1966 in the home of one of the social workers; the then-governor of Oregon, Mark Hatfield, lent us his Polaroid camera to record the event. That union, blessed by most of the professionals who had worked with both of us during our stay at the Cuckoo's Nest, defied all sensibilities, as did Mr. Kesey's story.

CHAPTER 14—THE HOLLY FAMILY

While I was trying to put my life back together at the mental hospital, my children were being shuffled from one foster home to another. Gardner, a strong-willed eleven-year-old, acted out the most. After three foster home placements failed, he was moved to St. Mary's Home for Boys in Beaverton.

At their first foster home, the children were all together, but it wasn't a good placement. The parents of that home didn't like Francis. He was always a timid child and he withdrew even deeper into his shell. Francis's bed was in the attic and he slept on a bare mattress because he was a bed wetter. When he continued to wet the bed he was forced to wear a dress.

The three youngest children were moved to a farm outside of Astoria, and Gardner went to live with their foster grandparents on a farm nearby. Danette, who was all of six years old, stood on a stool to wash dishes after each meal and again in the evening when she washed the milking equipment. Francis moved to another foster placement without Danette and Stephen who were placed together in the home of an older couple. Many of my letters to the children were never delivered to them, and the children's case workers found reasons to deny my requests for visit with the children.

When Dan retired, he went to Astoria. Although he was allowed some supervised visits with the children, the case workers claimed the visits were confusing for the children and made it difficult for the foster families. Dan went to court, and when he learned he couldn't take the children out of the state, he devised a screwball plan to bring a fishing boat up the Columbia, grab the children, and sail to Mexico. He left Oregon and headed to California after the failed attempt to visit me at the hospital. Although Oregon tried to collect child support; whenever they closed in on his trail, he moved on.

George did not want any part of step-parenting. I was promoted to a Secretary Two position at the state capitol, and was beginning to bring home a good paycheck. George, always the dreamer, decided we should buy a piece of land in the hills and build a cabin. He did find a couple who were willing to sell on contract, and without any credit we put $100 down and agreed to make monthly payments of $100 a month for two acres with river frontage. We put everything we owned in our old station wagon and moved onto our land to begin building a one-room cabin. On the first of each month, when his disability check arrived, we went to the lumberyard. We finished the cabin by Christmas and celebrated by stringing holiday lights across the front window. I cooked a turkey in an electric roaster. Although we had electricity, I still had to carry water from a spring. I bathed in the galvanized tub and pioneering was fun for awhile. Then the rain started in October, and by February cabin fever was killing me and our relationship. When I discovered mildew growing on the pictures of my children, I couldn't stay there any longer.

We sold the place as a vacation cabin and made a nice profit but I don't think George ever forgave me for wanting to move back to suburbia.

I wanted my children. George and I visited Gardner at a foster home in Beaverton and George agreed the situation was appalling. The foster mother was a large, burly woman who stacked boys in bunk beds in three bedrooms. She controlled the boys with obscenities and sometimes more than verbal abuse. When Gardner climbed a tree to avoid a beating, she forced him down by firing a gun into the air. George and I bought a small one-bedroom house with a shed in the back yard. We converted the shed into a cute bunkhouse and with the help of George's attorney we were able to gain custody of Gardner. He came home in June of 1967; a nervous twelve-year-old who wanted to believe that he was home for good.

Patty who had been writing to me sometimes was pregnant. I blamed myself and wanted to help her but George said, "You got one of your kids here, and that's it."

Gardner went to the fields to pick crops with other kids his age. Gardner was in and out of trouble with one farmer or the next and didn't make much money. Almost everything Gardner did aggravated George, who was drinking again that summer. George's rules for Gardner changed daily; depending on his mood he was either Gardner's defender or his accuser.

George and I were invited to go for a ride in the neighbor's new convertible; George wouldn't let Gardner come with us. When we got back, Gardner was jumping off a picnic table onto our dog. The dog had so many broken bones we had to put him down.

George made me take Gardner to the state hospital for an evaluation. Gardner and I went alone. He was small for his age, and he looked much younger than twelve that day as he sat on a chair in the doctor's office swinging his legs and smiling. I watched the black and white tennis shoes go back and forth, over and over, and I felt nauseated. Gardner was admitted to the hospital and he turned his face away when I tried to kiss him goodbye. He went with the attendant without looking back at me. I walked home with a heavy heart, hating my life again.

Gardner had a hard stay at the hospital. He fought every kind of treatment. Once when I went to visit him he was strapped to a bare mattress wearing only briefs. He was so heavily sedated his words were slurred and his eyes rolled up and sideways. After that I wasn't allowed to visit because they moved him to the secure unit. A little boy thrown in with the criminally insane! How could that have happened? The criminally insane person in our family was still sleeping in my bed.

Francis came home next. He had been placed with a family on the Oregon coast and the placement didn't work out. His case worker in Astoria called to ask me if I thought I was ready for a trial home placement with one of my children. My hungry, empty arms welcomed my seven-year-old son in spite of George's reluctance. The day that Francis arrived I took him to the Oregon State Fair. He held my hand and wouldn't ride on any of the rides if it meant he had to let go of my hand. He clung to me with a goofy smile and watched the merry-go-round and Ferris wheel while we ate cotton candy together. It was a wonderful day.

To soothe George's concern about another mouth to feed on his disability income, I went to work at a cannery, shoving ears of corn into a machine that tore the kernels off. I worked the night shift, and when Francis got up he watched TV while I slept. He never got dressed unless I made him. He just wanted to stay in the house with me for the rest of his life. With my first paycheck I bought him a pair of black galoshes with buckles across the front. He put them on first thing every morning, and would have worn them to bed if I hadn't stopped him.

When I enrolled Francis in school, I learned that Oregon had recently determined that children living in a home with a stepfather were still eligible for aid from the state. I was able get a welfare check and free cheese at the food bank. It didn't take long for George to do the math. He saw that we could get a bigger check and a lot of free food if we had all my children. He called his attorney to arrange for me to file for permanent custody of not only Francis, but Danette and Stephen too. Family Services in Astoria was reluctant to release the children. They saw a woman who had spent over a year in a mental hospital and then married another patient who had once been in the Astoria jail as a murder suspect.

At Halloween, I sewed a Batman outfit for Francis. We searched the rummage stores for tights and swimming trunks that I dyed the right colors. I made a cape, mask and even a tool belt for my little goblin. After a fun night of trick-or-treating, Francis wasn't ready to take the costume off. Everyday after school he became Batman and Francis didn't emerge until bedtime. He learned to sew enough to keep the tattered costume repaired until it finally fell apart. I was reminded of my Supergirl days back in the Brent Hotel when my mother was dying.

We moved to a larger house, and decorated the extra bedrooms for Danette and Stephen who would be joining us.

On Christmas Eve George drove us to Beaverton where we met the state car from Astoria to pick up the children. I didn't want to take a chance that Gardner might ruin Christmas morning for the fragile kids, so I went in the afternoon to pick bring him from the hospital. He opened his gifts after dinner, and he didn't seem to enjoy the gifts or the visit.

That winter wasn't a happy time for the any of us. Francis didn't want to share me and Danette who was almost ten and had learned about Jesus Christ in her foster home felt responsible for my salvation. Each night she read her Bible so loud in her bedroom upstairs that we had to turn up the volume on the television. Stephen didn't know me, and he kept crying for his mommy. Gardner was transferred to the boy's reform school in Woodburn where he promptly chewed the telephone cords in half because they wouldn't let him call me.

But we all began to adjust, even George who enjoyed the financial aid from the state. Danette and Francis were doing better in school, and although Stephen was old enough for kindergarten, I kept him home with me so we could get to know each other. He was a good boy and entertained himself for hours. I saved enough green stamps to buy him a wagon. He filled it with his favorite toys and pushed it around the sidewalk with one knee in the wagon. It disappeared from our front yard one day and we never found it. I couldn't afford to replace it. It was a pivotal loss for me. I hated George for not using some of the financial aid to buy Stephen a new wagon.

We qualified for HUD, which meant that our income was low enough to buy a subsidized house. The house was built according to a standard floor plan, but we got to pick out the colors. We moved in the day after Christmas. We began the new year with a home of our own. It should have been a wonderful new beginning for all of us, but George built a room in the garage and he deteriorated behind the locked door.

One morning my friend Kathy called from Montana. I couldn't understand what she was saying at first, and then I didn't want to believe what she was saying. Pierre, one of the twins that I had been so attached to, fell out of a pickup truck and died.

"Could I come for the funeral?"

I couldn't and I felt bad about not being able to be with her. George was again the reason for my unhappiness.

George was not financially responsible for my children, but he could have been emotionally supportive when I needed him most. Stephen was seriously injured while he and Francis were playing. A rusty nail hit Stephen in the eye. After a week in the hospital he was able to open both eyes, but he couldn't see out of the right one. George drove me to the hospital every day, but parked two blocks away so no one would see him. He was worried the hospital would expect him to pay the bill.

Later, George accused me of putting ground up glass in his sandwich and he started keeping his food in his garage room. He made a new rule that we could only buy brown bread. When he found a loaf of white bread in the refrigerator he accused me of defying his order. I wasn't able to convince him I had forgotten the bread rule. He took the loaf of bread to the back porch and began sailing the slices of bread into the yard like Frisbees. I laughed; he choked me until I passed out. After that I was afraid of him. I went to see a psychiatrist who knew both of us. I wanted George to move, but I didn't want to make him mad again. The doctor said it would be best if George thought it was his idea to move out. I didn't see how that could happen but thankfully it did.

George got a job at the cannery. He worked about three weeks before he announced he was leaving.

"This ain't my dream, Carol. This is your dream. I can't live like this working eight hours a day and coming home to a square box full of someone else's brats."

He had a white pickup and he pointed out that the children and I had a new house, welfare money and a dependable car and he was out of there. He laughed a sick little chuckle and said people would probably ask, "Who was that man who fixed up the widow lady and rode away on his white horse."

So the children and I were alone, and peace settled over our house for awhile. I went to work in a convenience store, and eventually advanced to manager. We struggled financially, but I was able to trade in our old jalopy for a new car. The sticker price was $1,999. 00 and I was so thankful that the dealership would sell me a car, I didn't even ask for a radio. We went on drives and went fishing on weekends. I was able to hang onto the car for over a year, but when 1973 was coming to an end, so was our budget. I sold it for what was left on the contract to protect my credit; and I rode a bicycle to work. It was dark when I left the house in the morning, and usually raining, so I kept a change of clothes at the store. When we needed groceries we all had to go so we could each carry a heavy sack home. After I bought Stephen a new wagon I made the shopping trip alone.

Francis got a paper route to help out, but he hated it. Every afternoon when the bundle was dropped in our driveway, he wailed while he prepared them for delivery. The neighbors knew their paper was coming soon. He made the same racket when he mowed the yard with our push lawnmower. One day he came home from his route sounding his misery from blocks away. He was carrying his bike in two pieces. The very old bike had broken in half; I let him quit the job.

Danette's friends lived in two-parent households and they could afford things we couldn't. Danette had a hard time dealing with that, but I was pleased that she had good friends and I wanted her to fit in, so I cut corners for her where I could. She was a great helper at home and a good second mother to her brothers, so she deserved a little extra.

Our life was hard but seemed to be getting better. Gardner came home for visits sometimes and Patty sent pictures of her two little girls. George filed for and paid for a divorce. I took back the name of Banich in 1973 and kept it for almost a year.

CHAPTER 15—THE LAPIN FAMILY

The kids and I were getting by. I was managing the store, and working evenings developing film. Some weekends I cooked hamburgers for a concession stand. We lived in a respectable neighborhood. We didn't have cockroaches or drunks in the bathtub, and we were had enough food to eat.

Danette found her niche in gymnastics and joined the drill team at school. At fourteen she was developing into the pretty young girl who would win Miss Physical Fitness in the 1976 Miss Oregon pageant. Gardner, still at the boys' school came home for visits and he was working toward a parole. The boys, Francis and Stephen, were in Scouts. They had a shaggy dog name Jake that they shared their room with. But I was alone. I felt incomplete without a husband. I dated a couple of men, but one was married, and the other one was too young.

I took a part-time job at a tavern on the edge of town, and learned to play pool. I began spending too much time in the bar away from my children. I met a guy at the bar who had never been married and seemed kinda shy. He lived on a farm where he helped his mother care for his dad who had multiple sclerosis. Even when he had drowned his inhibitions in beer he blushed when we made eye contact. Our first date, if you could call it that, was at the fire station. I was locking up the bar and Frank was pretty drunk, so I drove him over to the station. As captain of the volunteer fire department Frank had a sleeping room there. He was too drunk to blush that night, and also too drunk to do anything but sleep after we crawled in together, but we began dating after that. He introduced me to water skiing, and we went horse back riding on the farm. We drank together and enjoyed each other, but we didn't have a sexual relationship. I thought I had finally found a man who wanted to be with me for something other than sex. Frank was a nice-looking guy with dark blond hair and a ruddy complexion. His broad face widened even more in a great smile.

Frank invited the children and me to the Lapin family's annual Labor Day Corn Feed. Each year his family invited friends and neighbors to join them in a harvest celebration. The event included swimming in the pool, riding horses, live music and lots to eat. No one was more surprised than I when, after the right amount of beer, Frank announced that we would be getting married in the spring!

Sometimes Frank seemed withdrawn and secretive. I worried about that side of him, and I asked one of our friends about it. He hesitated before he drawled, "Well, maybe Frank just isn't the marrying kind."

When I pressed for an explanation, he said, "Be careful."

Careful! When had I ever been careful? What I saw was a handsome young man who treated me special, and didn't take advantage of me sexually. We would have a home in the country with a swimming pool. My children would be able to go boating and water skiing, ride a motor cycle and even have a horse of their own.

I traded my house for a trailer that we set up on the farm, and I married Frank in the spring of 1974 in a small ceremony at a Lutheran Church. We honeymooned on the Oregon coast; Frank was drunk most of that time.

We settled into married life. Frank had a large following of young boys, partly because of the boat, and partly because he provided the beer they were too young to buy. He owned a lot in a recreational park in the mountains where he had set up an old camp trailer. On weekends campers gathered around their fires in the evening and people visited back and forth. Of course there was a lot of drinking at the camp too. My kids loved to go to the camp, especially if the boat was going too, but Frank left us home some weekends. I was always disappointed, but I tried to understand that Frank needed "guy" time with his friends.

Francis was sick a lot, and was missing too much school. He had flu-like symptoms and began losing weight. Frank's mother said she thought he had the "yaller jawness." Our doctor thought Francis was having some emotional problems. He put him on a tranquilizer, and recommended Maalox for his other problems.

Frank wanted to adopt my boys and we talked with Francis and Stephen about that. Both boys liked the idea, so we started the adoption process. Francis wanted to change his first name to Frank, which would make him Frank Lapin, Jr.

Gardner was paroled and he married a young girl he had been dating on home visits. They lived with her parents. Nancy—pretty, quiet, and smitten with Gardner—was soon pregnant. Gardner's red hair had darkened to mahogany and his freckles had faded some. Not only was he good looking, he had the charm of a graduate con. Shortly after the baby was born in 1974, Gardner went to prison for car theft. I talked with Nancy and told her how hard my life had been. I encouraged her to take the baby away and start over. I did not see baby Shane again until he was thirty-one years old.

When I joined the Marion County Volunteer Fire Department I was the first female volunteer. What I really wanted to do was work on the ambulance as an EMT, but I had to be a member of the fire department for that training. Once a week I reported to the fire station for training and practice exercises. I kept my place and didn't try to compete with the guys and they began to accept me. That was when my initiation began. Not one of them explained that I should always hold onto the top bar while standing on the running board of the truck; then when we bounced over railroad tracks I wouldn't loose my grip when I flew into the air. But I hung on, literally, and I learned to bend my knees slightly to absorb the shock of the road. Then I studied the manual and learned how to operate the hydraulic controls on the pumper truck. That was something I could do. I couldn't manage a hose full of pressurized water. I could also drive the truck as well as a guy, expect for the time I arrive first and pulled the truck out of the station alone. I was two blocks away from the fire when the truck froze up. The emergency lights were flashing and the siren was on and so were the emergency brakes.

Frank and I were featured in the Statesman Journal when he was named fireman of the year and I took the trophy for rookie of the year.

We were a team everywhere, except in the marital bed. Frank simply did not want to have sex with me. When I found him sleeping in the boys' beds some mornings, I figured he had come home drunk and hadn't wanted to risk having to say no again.

One weekend his mother, the kids, and I drove up to the campground for the weekend. Frank had gone up earlier with one of the guys who worked at the gas station with him. It was late when we pulled into the lot; the campfires were out, and none of the campers were around. When I opened the door to the camper I saw Frank and his friend in the bed, curled up together, and naked. I shut the door before his mother could see. I told her Frank was passed out drunk, and I wanted to go back to town. She asked a few questions, but barely protested. I wondered if she knew.

When Frank came back to town he made a big display of pouring all his alcohol down the sink and promising never to drink again. Of course, that didn't last long. Even after I had been slapped in the face with Frank's sexual encounter with his friend I didn't think about any risk for my sons. I told myself Frank had been so drunk he hadn't known what he was doing.

One of our tavern friends, Sydney, had purchased a brand new 280Z car, and was showing it to Frank's relatives when I went across the street to borrow a cigarette. Sydney said he won a sales contest at work and had two tickets to Hawaii, but he had no one to go with. I said, "Hell, I'll go with you."

"Frank ain't going to let you go to Hawaii with me," he laughed.

But Frank's aunt told him Frank probably would let me go, and one thing led to another. After a couple of beers and a lot of laughing I bet Sydney $100 that Frank would say I could go.

The next morning I told Frank about the bet. I told him I would give him $50 if he would call Sydney up and tell him it was all right with him if I went to Hawaii. He did, and I went to Hawaii with Sydney. By the time we came back, I knew I would leave Frank and move in with Sydney. The boys didn't want to leave the farm, and Danette announced she would move in with her girlfriend across the street.

I denied everything I felt and knew and left my sons on the farm. The price for that mistake was way too high for any mother to ever pay.

CHAPTER 16—THE HOLOBOFFS

(Sydney) Sergie Nickoliovich Holoboff's ancestors escaped the pogroms in Russia in the 1800s and fled to Canada. His parents left their communal Dukabor life in Saskatchewan and came to the United States during the worst of the Great Depression. Mary was pregnant with her third child, Wasili, who we call William. Her husband Nick earned enough bounty rewards from killing prairie dogs to load what little the family owned into a rattletrap car. Sydney's sisters, Molly and Polly, crammed into the back seat between boxes, looked like their mother with the same colorful dresses and babushkas.

Nick and Mary took any work they could find. They picked hops, berries, and beans, and they cleaned turkey carcasses at a plant where they tied the youngest child to a table in the lunch room. They dressed their children in free Salvation Army clothes, and by the time Sydney was born in 1940, Molly was taking over at home while Mary, with a lot more drive and ambition than Nick, worked wherever she could. They socked away dollars to buy a house, and then they moved one more time to the farmhouse they were living in thirty-five years later when I arrived on the scene.

The Holoboffs, including the children, planted rows of boysenberries and strawberries on their forty acres, and they also worked for other farmers in the area. They bought more land every chance they could, and as the fertile Willamette Valley land increased in value and subdivisions grew where there had once been crops, those crazy Russians—as their neighbors called them—turned their sock money into millions.

The older children were married and raising families of their own by the time Sydney finished high school. He worked as a carpenter's helper, but then a neighbor, nursing a broken leg, hired him as a chauffeur. Sydney drove to grain elevators all over the northwest where the neighbor maintained scales that weighed grain before it was loaded into boxcars. Sydney learned the trade, and when his mentor retired, Sydney bought the franchise and incorporated what he called Northwest Automatic Scales.

Sydney, the baby of the family, was spoiled as most last children are. He didn't have to work as hard as his sisters and brother, but there were very few carefree childhood memories for any of them. They were teased and called Communists during the Cold War years. Sydney remembers only one toy, a wooden dog on wheels that he pulled around behind him. Sometimes the entire family stopped working early and went into the house to watch the Three Stooges, or they went swimming in the reservoir after supper. Nick and Mary dropped the kids off in a secluded area to climb over the fence to get into the state fair at Salem. Mary, with only one year of schooling, was illiterate and although Nick went no further than fifth grade, he could read well enough to distort "Anna Ladder's" advice column. When he read the newspaper to Mary he changed the columnist's answers to suit himself and in fact, most of what Mary knew about the world was Nick's distorted version. She developed diabetes and when the nurse gave her a diet to follow, Mary pretended she could read. I discovered she was injecting saline from the practice bottle the nurse gave her because she didn't want to open the new vial—which was insulin— until she used all the free medicine.

Mary's only handicap was illiteracy. Had she been educated, she would have been unstoppable. She could study a doily briefly in the Ben Franklin store, then go home and replicate the pattern with her crochet hook.

Their two-story farmhouse, always in need of repair and updating, received occasional facelifts with paint and wallpaper, or another used oil-stove replaced an old one. They rarely used the indoor plumbing. Every time I visited, they blamed me for plugging up the old septic tank. They used the odd house—their word for the privy in the back yard. A rotten walnut-tree fell on it once but Nick had the boys dig a new hole; they dragged the old two-seater to the fresh pit.

Nick and Mary had several Russian friends and on weekends, after borsch, when their glasses were filled with vodka, they gathered around the kitchen table and sang a Capella late into the night.

The family spoke Russian at home. Sydney didn't start school until he was seven, and then he had to repeat the first grade because of his language barrier. He was nine years old when he was promoted to the second grade.

Sydney was terribly shy until he had a few drinks, but unlike Frank he was very interested in me sexually and at times he embarrassed me. He wore western-style suits with embroidered yokes, cowboy boots, and a bolo tie that look like a noose around his thick neck. While I was at work, he was sleeping until noon. After he showered in the banya—a steam-bath shed at the farm—he used too much aftershave. He combed his hair with hair oil and his fine hair separated into individual strands. He waited for me in front of the building where I worked in his fancy car. There he would be, puffing on a fat cigar; when he saw me he yelled, "Hi ya honey!"

We went out to eat every night of the week, and every night of the week ended with sex. To make sure I would be there when he needed me, Sydney hired me as an assistant and traveling companion.

He was the only automatic scale technician west of the Mississippi, and that made me the only female scale technician anywhere. He sold, maintained and rebuilt automatic dump scales scattered across the Dakotas, Montana, Idaho, Washington and Oregon.

Most of the automatic scales are in the cupola of grain elevators; ninety or more feet above the ground. There are several ways to get to the cupola. I found the outside climb the scariest, even with the ladder in a safety cage. The ladders inside the elevators were in a narrow dark space and they were so old I had to test each rotting board. Spider webs brushed across my face and by the time I could see daylight from above I was often in tears. Sometimes we used a manlift with heavy pulley ropes that passed through a wooden platform. To lift the platform, we had to pull on the ropes and release a foot peddle to stop it. It was hard not to come down too fast if there was a lot of weight on the platform. The machinery required no oil or lubrication if I did my job properly. I scraped the metal couplings with a pocket knife until they moved smoothly without any friction.

Sydney, who had no fear of heights, dangled his feet out the elevator loft while we ate his lunch. I kept my distance but I risked both our lives by smoking in the combustible elevator dust. We took advantage of the private high-rise workplace in other ways too.

Sydney wanted a family, at least the one male child he had promised his mother he would have. The Holoboffs had five granddaughters, but in their mind, no heirs. Sydney kept asking me to see if a doctor could fix my tubes. I was sure that was impossible and I thought he might not want me if I couldn't have a child. I found a doctor who thought he could repair my tubes could be reattached, though he said it would be experimental but he was more concerned about my mental stability when he learned I had been sterilized at the state hospital. He asked where my children were and I lied and said they were all living with me and doing well. He told me he was going to think about the situation and check the references I had given him.

While Sydney was not the proverbial handsome prince, there were many reasons that I was ready to get married for the fifth time. His family was old fashioned and stable; the Holoboff family had never had a divorce. This man had pursued me; for the first time I was the lovee instead of the lover. I wanted a home, and most of all I wanted another baby. Francis and I talked about my plans to marry Sydney and he told me he didn't want another stepfather. I told Francis I was tired of being poor and I wanted to give my kids the things I thought they deserved; maybe they could go to a private prep school and college.

I had the operation to repair my tubes in September, shortly after my divorce from Frank became final. Ironically, when I came out of the anesthetic I found a teddy-bear frog on my bed with a card around its neck that read, "From the handsome prince."

While I was in the hospital, surrounded by flowers and gifts, Danette won the Miss Physical Fitness award in the Miss Oregon pageant. My absence at that event was just one of the many things that drove a long lasting wedge between us.

The wedding date was set for December 11th. When Sydney bought a piano for my wedding gift, Mary and Nick, who were in the kitchen when it was delivered, pointed and shouted in Russian. Sydney and I didn't even have a bed of our own.

The first time I had a hint I had of Sydney's emotional instability—or maybe it was the first time I couldn't blame his behavior on alcohol—Sydney and I were going out on a last job site before the wedding and we had the invitations addressed and stamped. He was pouting because he had to wait for me to heal from the surgery. He told his Dad not to mail the invitations because he wasn't sure anymore. I cried halfway across Idaho before he said everything was all right. He called his dad that night and the invitations went out as planned.

I was embarrassed to be planning such a lavish wedding ceremony for my fifth time up the aisle. But Sydney had never been married, and the Methodist minister said that in a public ceremony, the promises we would make to each other would also be made to people who were important to us. Danette was my bridesmaid. She walked ahead of me and Francis and Stephen were both at my side as we walked past the many friends and relatives who came to celebrate with us. The three of them handed me off to Sydney when we reached the altar. Sydney had his dream wedding and a large reception too. Mary and several of her Russian friends served borscht to over 300 people who also went through a buffet line. As is customary at a Russian wedding, Sydney and I filled silly requests made by the guests and they gave us money to start our new life. When an elderly friend of the family told Sydney that he was gaining quite a family and he said the children wouldn't be living with us, she told him not to be too sure. She was right, even though that night, after Frank filled up on Nick's free booze, my boys went home with him.

We honeymooned in the South Pacific. Although it sounds like something out of a fairytale, it was actually out of a National Geographic. Sydney had been to Fiji and when he read about the Truk harbor, where the United States sunk so many Japanese ships, he chose that island for our honeymoon.

From the minute the stewardess leaned over our seat to remind us that we were on a family flight, to the return flight when lightning struck our plane, the honeymoon was a nightmare for me. I hate flying, even under the best of circumstances, but the landing strips on the islands were frequently just large pieces of coral. The 737 jumbo jet braked hard immediately at touchdown and stopped with its nose protruding over water on the other side of the island.

My groom was drunk for most of the honeymoon; although there weren't any snakes in paradise there were dinner-plate-size garden spiders. Sydney passed out the night I encountered one of the colorful, hairy-legged, harmless spiders in the bathroom of our grass-hut.

It was Christmas, and I was homesick for my children. Sydney saw my sadness as a rejection of him. He threw an engraved gold-plated lighter he had given me into the harbor. Only after I had cried enough to convince him that I loved him, did he show me that he hadn't really thrown it. That was the same groom who paid extra for the restaurant to order some chocolate from Hawaii for me and the same tender husband who brought me breakfast in bed, and let me win at crazy eights.

Francis came to the farm visibly upset just a few days after we returned from our honeymoon. I could tell he had been crying and he said Frank was going to put Stephen in a foster home. I said that would never happen! Sydney knew when I told Francis I was going to stop the adoption and that he and his brother were going to live with us, that there was no turning back. I have never seen a teenage boy sob like Francis did that day. He put his head in his arms on the table and cried with his entire body. Sydney and I were unable to calm him and I was crying with Francis. I hadn't suspected that he was so unhappy at Frank's; and in fact it would be years before I understood the depth of his relief to be free of Frank.

Sydney hired an attorney and I told him about drugs that Frank left in secret places for his teenaged friends. The adoptions, not finalized, were annulled. When Sydney and I went to Frank's to pick up the boys they were in the driveway with all of their possessions, even the light bulbs from their bedrooms. That night I welcomed my sons with a warm fire and clean beds. When Nick and Mary came home from their winter vacation in New Zealand, they found my family living there.

Step parenting came hard for Sydney. He tried to set rules about homework and table manners to two half-grown boys, who had been left to their own devices during their formative years. Francis tried hard to please Sydney, but Stephen's response was anger. And so was mine. It was overwhelming to try to keep the peace between my new husband and my sons, and I was pregnant!

Sydney and I had an argument one afternoon and when I ran upstairs crying Mary followed me. She said, "Sydney is mean sometimes. How you going to live with him?"

I swiped my sleeve across my face and told her I would have to figure it out because we were going to have a baby. Her response to that was a sorrowful, "Oh, no."

When Sydney found out that I had told his mother I was pregnant, he was furious. He said that I should get an abortion.

"I wanted to tell my parents about the baby!"

When I responded to his cruel suggestion by throwing a kitchen chair at him, the mood was broken when his father cried out: "Oy! Be careful. You'll break my chair." We all laughed and finally recognized the miracle of my pregnancy.

Sydney, the boys and I moved into a townhouse in an exclusive golf club resort, and set up a bank account for Danette so she could have her own apartment until she finished high school. I had an amniocentesis; the baby was healthy. But about the same time that we were celebrating that good news, Francis began having flu-like symptoms again.

One morning when he claimed to be too tired to go to school, Sydney said he was going to find out once and for all if Francis was really sick. He made an appointment for Francis with his family doctor. The day the results of Francis's blood work came back the doctor called me at home and asked me to bring Francis back for more tests. The next day he was admitted to the hospital. The tests he had while he was there included a painful bone marrow and a liver biopsy. Within a week, we learned Francis had non-A, non-B hepatitis, and that he had extensive liver damage. We were advised to send Francis back to school and encourage him to live his life as normally as possible. The doctor said, "Who knows? Maybe someday we will be able to do liver transplants."

Sydney never accepted the strong possibility that Francis would die; I feared that each day might be his last. If he didn't wake up in time for school, if he didn't come home from school right away, if he fell down, if he threw up, my anxiety increased. Francis agreed with Sydney that I was just being a worrywart mother, and he frequently told me to leave him alone.

I loved being pregnancy. I cried happy tears for the future when I felt my baby moving, and then I cried sad tears for Francis's uncertain future.

Danette had been dating a young deputy sheriff and when they came to show us her engagement ring I thought it was the first time I had seen her really happy for many years. I went to the hospital in October to have the baby, Francis and Stephen stayed with Danette, and for that short time our family seemed normal and happy.

Pascha Sergeiovich (son of Sergei) Holoboff was born on October 15, 1977 by emergency C-section. Sydney had produced the male heir for the Holoboffs; he partied hard with family and friends and showered me with flowers and jewelry until the day before I left the hospital.

Sydney came to the hospital in a foul mood. I eventually coaxed the reason for his misery out of him. His mother told him I would probably leave him now that I had the baby. I went into my little woman act, crying to assure him I would never leave him or take his little boy away. He recovered from his morose mood before we brought our bundle of joy home.

Pascha was not an easy baby. He cried with colic almost every day. Stephen announced he would never hold the baby, and Francis couldn't hold his baby brother enough. Sydney was not sure how he felt about sharing me with his son; he was especially jealous when I nursed him. Danette loved holding the baby and shopping for tiny clothes.

I thought he was a beautiful infant, but Sydney didn't want to purchase the newborn pictures because he said Pascha was the ugliest baby he had ever seen and he didn't want the pictures hanging in our house. Sydney's sister Molly said she thought he was real cute and added, "He doesn't have your big nose."

But it wasn't his little scrunched up frown and fuzzy round head that I fell in love with. It was his velvet skin and his new baby smell and his nuzzles at my breast as he sought to connect. Every dream that I had had for my other children, dreams that had died because of others and sometimes because of me, I wrapped around that little boy. He would have a good life.

Patty married Greg in December and he brought his little girl Wendy into the family. We traveled with our boys to Spokane for the ceremony. Pascha cried during the ceremony and the reception but Patty just laughed and told everyone the screaming infant in the cloak room was another brother. Between Shirley and me, Patty had six brothers and two sisters.

Danette didn't laugh when Pascha screamed through her wedding and reception in January and I had to admit that "Little Lord Fauntleroy" in his wine-colored velvet romper and lace bib nearly ruined the day for Danette and Dan. Sydney didn't go back to work until Pascha was six months old. He used all of our savings. He was afraid to miss minute of his boy's development. We have pictures of Pascha's "first" everything. There wasn't the large amount of money I had been led to believe and Sydney was beginning to realize that the "hotty" he thought he had married didn't like sex all that much. The stepsons were more than he had bargained for, and his baby screamed all the time. Gardner was paroled and looking for a home; Sydney made it clear, in a loud, profane way that he was not taking in anymore of my kids. If I wanted to see Gardner, I could go to a café to visit him. Gardner went to live with Frank for a short while, and then in a stolen car crossed the state line in search of his Banich dad.

Sydney said, and he said it many more times over the years, no matter where we were living, "I'm getting the hell out of this town!"

He finally worked up enough steam to take action, and we moved to Montana and he went back to work. Sydney's moods fluctuated with the balance in his checkbook.

We rented a duplex in Great Falls in the spring of 1978, and callously yanked the boys out of school in the middle of the term. Francis, in his junior year of high school, adjusted to the move by joining a chess club and the Boy Scout Explorer program. He wanted to be a policeman, so he went into the Junior Deputy Sheriff Unit. The other love of Francis's life was our maroon pickup. Sydney let him drive it once in a while; when Francis wasn't driving it, he was washing it

Stephen continued to defy every rule that Sydney made. When Stephen refused to turn out the light in his bedroom, Sydney put a ten-watt bulb in the lamp; Stephen silently lived with the change. When he refused to empty the trash in his room, Sydney grounded him for a week; Stephen stayed home without a whimper.

Stephen had a paper route that first winter. He came home some mornings with ice on his lips from his runny nose and frostbitten toes, but he was faithful about getting papers to his customers. However, he was too shy to collect payments from the deadbeats on his route, so he didn't make much money.

My friend Kathleen plugged in her coffee pot and we picked up our friendship as though I had never left town. Her granddaughter was just six months younger than Pascha so we shopped with them in strollers and stepped over their toys just as though we were back in the 50's.

Margaret came to visit and fussed over Pascha and expressed surprise over how big the boys were, but her mission was clearly in her purse. She brought bank statements and records from my mother's savings account. She was concerned that I might have thought she spent my college money. I almost refused to look at the papers, but I finally pretended to; I didn't want to know. After that first visit we included my sister in our holiday and birthday celebrations, but I always felt there that there was something keeping her from really enjoying our relationship.

On the surface my life seemed to be all that I had ever hoped for. But when the boys were in school, I took Pascha to a nearby park and while I pushed him in the swing, I cried. I cried for Francis, I cried for Stephen who deserved more than he was getting from his stepfather, but mostly I cried for Pascha. I don't know why I thought I could bring my own emotional problems to a partnership with an insecure, immature, alcoholic, and expect to find Norman Rockwell. I was wanted Pascha to grow up in a good two-parent home.

Stephen got caught for shoplifting and we had to go to counseling. Sydney went to the sessions hoping he could convince me and the counselor to put Stephen in a foster home or boy's school. As the sessions went on it became clear that Stephen was the sacrificial lamb at our house. He was taking abuse from Sydney for Francis or me. I didn't see that until Sydney refused to go to an appointment and Stephen and I went alone. The counselor asked, "Where's—" and before he could say Sydney I snarled, "You mean the asshole?"

There was a few seconds of silence, then he said, "You know, I always suspected the issues were not about Stephen. What's really going on?"

He sent Stephen out of the room and for the first time in two years, I talked about the mess I had created. I poured out my frustrations. I talked about the guilt I felt about deceiving Sydney and my determination to make the best of it. I told him about Sydney's sexual demands and the retaliations he had made when they were not met. I said that Sydney and I had gone to a psychiatrist twice, but when nothing changed in the bedroom Sydney refused to go back.

After that Stephen didn't go with us to counseling. The therapist referred Sydney and me to another counselor. He advised me to tell Sydney the doctor specialized in marriage problems. Sydney went with me a couple of times; when he stopped going, I went alone.

Dr. Taylor only half kidding, told me it was hard for Sydney and me to communicate because Sydney's goals were in his balls and mine were in my head. I saw Dr. Taylor every week for almost a year. He asked me to journal my thoughts during the week and to bring the journal to our sessions. It was the first time I had looked in my own soul and with his wise mentoring I began to know who I was then, who I had been, and most importantly who I wanted to be. He said although I was becoming insightful and introspective, I had not really found myself yet. Dr. Taylor told me I was a virtuous woman but he still had to explain that had nothing to do with virginity. He showed me the dictionary definitions: good, righteous, worthy, honorable, moral, upright, and honest. Was I really any of those things? I doubted it then but the seed was planted.

Dr. Taylor accused me of just waiting around for the next funeral and I began to see that he was right. I was afraid to live. I had learned how to live with death, but I hadn't learned how to live with people and because Dr. Taylor believed I could, I began to try.

I supported Francis in his decision to move back to Oregon after his graduation. Then in a drunken rage, Sydney beat Stephen with his fists. Stephen bought a bus ticket, packed his things in a box, and when he came into the living room he said; "I'm leaving. You'll never see me again. Do you have anything you want to say?"

I, the virtuous, introspective, insightful, woman of therapy, said nothing. He left home the day before Thanksgiving in 1981, and I cried a long time, but it would be a long time before I cried again. Sydney's sister called to say she had seen Stephen at a store in Salem, so at least I knew he was in Oregon

Then it was just Sydney, three-year-old-Pascha and me. There were no scapegoats, no buffers. I continued to see my therapist, and began to believe in my possibilities. He helped me recognize my talents and strengths and I realized I had developed many survival skills during my tumultuous life. Although Dr. Taylor never encouraged me to leave Sydney he did help me examine my pathological dependence on men. I saw that I had gone from one bad relationship to another, over and over. I hadn't learned from my mistakes, and foolishly expected different outcomes from the same behaviors.

The day I realized I hadn't found a handsome prince, but just another drunken frog, my sadness and self-pity turned to rage! My anger brought me out of the helpless victim role, and gave me the strength to make changes. Sydney's business was in financial ruin, he hadn't filed taxes for two years. I told him that I was worried about our finances, and that I was going to move back to Oregon, go to school and then to work. I don't know which one of us was more surprised at the calm way he listened to my plans. I guess I thought he would blow a gasket, but he seemed almost relieved. I packed, just for Pascha and me. Sydney loaded our furniture in a U-haul truck and his brother helped him unload the furniture into an apartment in Salem, Oregon. Then Sydney went back to Great Falls until the lease on the house was up.

While he was living alone he woke up one morning with a huge hematoma over his eye and he couldn't remember driving after he left a bar thirty miles out of Great Falls the night before. He later told me that he got down on his knees that day and promised God he would never take another drink. He never did. Not even communion wine.

CHAPTER 17—COMING OUT OF CHUTE #2

During my psychotherapy I began to wonder what became of the youngest cowgirl in Montana. What had happened to that wild child who believed she could ride to the moon and back? When did she stop believing?

Empowered by years of suppressed anger that was finding a voice, I was ready to try again. I planned to grab hold with both hands and I planned to finish the ride. I wouldn't need to wave a white hat to reassure the crowd. Fuck the crowd!

White-hot anger burned in my gut and spewed out in eruptions of rage that rained equally on the innocent and the guilty. When the venomous contents were spent, silent dry heaves were my private companions.

Freedom's just another word for nothing left to lose; a line from Me and Bobby McGee became my mantra. I mentally bound my baby boy for the sacrifice. Pascha was all that stood between Mrs. Sydney Holoboff and Carol D. Johnson. Everything else was dispensable. I was prepared to move into a shopping cart under the bridge if necessary. Never again, I vowed, would I let anyone take advantage of me, abuse me, torment me or make me say I loved them. This body was not lying down for another climactic Academy Award performance.

A career counselor at the community college may have seen a young woman dressed in a housedress and wearing anklets and snickered when he helped me arrange to take the SAT (Scholastic Aptitude Test) required of all college-bound students. I was dressed in the same desperate housewife attire when the same counselor discovered I had scored high in the test; in the 99.5 percentile.

"That is quite an achievement for someone who dropped out of high school years ago," he offered, "but I'm afraid you will find the science courses required for a nursing degree overwhelming. You might consider enrolling in the nurse's aide program instead."

I hadn't taken the class on assertiveness yet and I lit into him.

"What Goddamn right do you have to discourage me from entering the nursing program? How the hell do you know what I can or cannot do? You probably told your wife she couldn't buy white bread, you son-of-a-bitch!"

He had no idea where that had come from, and I didn't try to explain.

"I don't care how you handle it," I shouted at Sydney. "I'm going to school this fall, and I guess that means you or someone else will have to take care of the kid."

I threw dishes at Sydney; he ducked. He chased me with hunks of firewood; I ran. "No wife of mine is going to work," he sputtered through clenched teeth.

"Tell that to Pascha's stepmother that when you find one," I yelled back.

The week before classes were to start, I went to the campus with my schedule in my hand and walked the halls until I knew exactly where each class was. I was the only one who knew how frightened I was the first day. My vision was fuzzy due to my high anxiety, I was afraid I might pass out on the steps of the main building.

For the next five years, until I had my Bachelor of Science degree in Nursing in my hand, I lived in fear that someone would find out I was an imposter. I struggled with chemistry and algebra; I hadn't had those classes in high school. In 1954 girls could substitute home economics classes for science, so I had learned how to can peaches instead.

As I approached menopause I was trying to grasp braces and brackets and equations and symbols. Sydney hired a tutor and I dropped beginning algebra and started over. I finished the class with an A, going on to advanced algebra easily. I decided algebra was a lot like doing push-ups; and I would need a well-toned brain for the next few years.

In September of 1983, in my 45th year, I was ready for the rodeo. I stepped up to the challenge of nursing school. I was surprised that nursing professors ate their young and that they couldn't see the correlation between the methods they used to teach nursing students and the nursing shortages. I felt that if I could grit my teeth and learn to curtsy I might make it through the fall term and receive my Nurses' Aide certificate, but it was a struggle for to keep my place without feeling like I was compromising my newfound dignity. My nursing class was drilled, in military fashion, to do and not ask why. A student might be sent home for the day because the nursing instructor found a wrinkle in the bed during skills lab. If that student cried, she might be labeled emotionally unstable. God help me—I thought to myself—if any of those instructors find out I was in the state hospital. One instructor who had a reputation of tormenting nursing students for the fun of it, decided to push my buttons one day; I think just to see what kind of music I would make. She stopped me in the hall at the hospital where I was doing a clinical rotation, leaned close to me and said; "I don't know why you keep coming back to class. You're never going to be a real nurse."

I pointed my finger at her face and told her, "Don't you ever talk to me again without a witness!"

Then I ran out of the hospital, got in my car and when I regained my composure I drove to the campus. I was afraid that I had kicked my opportunity for a better life in the face. I went to the dean of nursing, and I told her had happened and how I felt that nursing instructor was harming the entire program. I showed her the briefcase I was carrying and claimed it held months of documentation about the instructor's interactions with, not just me, but also many of the nursing students. Then I dug into my gambling genes and risked it all when I told the dean that I could not train under that instructor one more day and if it meant I would have to drop out of program I would. I told her I would be contacting an attorney.

There was nothing in the briefcase, but I had something else much more valuable; support from my peers. I began getting calls from former nursing students who had trained under that same instructor; they were willing to come forward. The attorney began talking about a class action suit. I didn't think I would be allowed to continue in the nursing program, but it turned out much different. Not only did I continue with my class, I gained the respect of the other nursing instructors and the friendship of fellow students. The instructor left the campus and later lost her professional license, not because of what she had done to me, but because I brought her actions to the attention of the right people.

No doubt Sydney was the recipient of my displaced anger. I bombarded him with verbal cruelty that should have been delivered to Dan for deserting us or George who made me to put Gardner in the state hospital or Frank who I was beginning to believe did the most damage of all to my sons. I screamed at Sydney when he did anything that reminded me of what the others had done. Our roles were reversing. I was becoming the abuser and Sydney the victim. But Sydney was growing too. He decided to be baptized in the Methodist Church and continued his vow of abstinence. He seemed almost relieved that someone had finally said STOP! He paid my tuition, and enrolled Paschal in a Montessori center. Sydney was vicariously sharing the fun of seeing my name on the honor roll in the newspaper and before long he was enmeshed in my activities. What had started as my rebellion became our coalition.

Stephen started coming over to visit. Danette and Dan had a daughter close to Pascha's age and we made Halloween outfits for our little ones. Francis and Stephen took them trick-or-treating, and made sure they collected enough candy for the winter. Danette's family and Francis stayed overnight with us on Christmas and Stephen came for dinner. Both Patty and Gardner called with holiday greetings.

The Holoboff family was healing. We had made a quantum leap. I welcomed 1984 with a silent toast; "out with the old and in with the new."

Nick and Mary, and Sydney and the kids clapped wildly and whistled when I was capped at the LPN graduation ceremony in May. I had been accepted into the Oregon Health Science University's bachelor of nursing program and I planned to commute to Portland in the fall. Sydney and Pascha would batch during the week and I would come home for the weekend. My first nursing job was at a nursing home. Every nurse can tell you a horror stories about her first job. But I took my nemesis to work with me; the instructor from hell, who might have destroyed my dreams. I felt her hovering above like a specter, waiting for me to screw up. And I did. I gave the wrong medicine to a patient. I freaked out and called the administrator at her home, hysterically reporting my error. When she discovered the medication I had given to the wrong patient was a multi-vitamin, she was kind enough not to laugh. Another evening I went to work with a severe migraine. I was working at the medication cart dispensing medicine in paper cups to the patients. Suddenly, without warning, I vomited a projectile stream all over the cart. The administrator was not laughing when she had to come in and order another cart from the pharmacy. She sent me home where I stayed, humiliated, and fearing I had permanently ruined my career as a nurse.

I was successful at my next nursing job. Pascha and I went to a summer camp in the country where I worked as camp nurse for the deaf campers. We stayed seven weeks. Pascha, who lived in a cabin with other seven-year-olds, quickly learned to sign.

One day that fall after Pascha was settled in school, and I was getting ready to leave for dormitory life, I woke up in the middle of the night to very loud pounding on my door. I opened just a little to see who was there and I saw it was Francis, holding a bloody towel to his face.

"My nose started bleeding and I can't make it quit," he told me.

I put a cold compress on his neck and showed him how to pinch his nose while I got dressed. When I came back into the front room, I found him on the back porch. He was vomiting and there was blood in the flower bed. My hand was shaking so much that I could hardly get the car keys into the ignition. The receptionist at the emergency room pushed through the double doors and attendants came running with a stretcher. The doctors in Salem weren't able stop the steady trickle that seemed like a geyser to me. Francis and I went by ambulance to the university hospital in Portland. I was frozen in prayer during the forty mile ride.

Francis had been taking quinine for very painful cramps in his legs; he had a reaction to that medicine that destroyed his platelets and his blood would not clot. No matter how many blood or platelet infusions the doctors gave Francis, it looked like he would bleed to death. Sydney and I went to his apartment to get a few personal items for him. Francis had a collection of survival clothes and equipment; that day there was drops of blood on everything. I cried at the irony of bloody survival items. We breathed a little when his platelet count rose above 1,000, even though the normal level is around 300,000. When the urine in the bag hanging on Francis' bed faded to pink, and then to dark orange, we toasted survival with orange juice and laughed at the gods. That crisis passed and Francis became eligible for employee health insurance, which meant he might be able to pay for a liver transplant, which doctors were doing with some success by then.

The next time Francis pounded on my front door, he shook with happy excitement. He had purchased a brand new truck, his first and only.

"You did not buy that," I challenged. "I bet you are just trying it out."

"No! Honest, Mom, it's all mine. Come on, I'll take you for a spin."

Tears stayed in my happy heart but not on my face that day when Francis drove me around in his new truck.

I was frightened about entering a university to study for my bachelor's degree in nursing and I knew as I drove around the winding Terwilliger Drive in southwest Portland that I was entering unknown territory and an unknown future. I was equally certain that there was no turning back. The university campus, old brick and stone buildings and high-rise medical towers, was large and formidable. In my new world there were libraries with something called stacks, and there were students from all over the world. Medical students, dental students, nursing students, and me!

The dorm was coed, but the nurse's floor was mostly girls. I felt uneasy when I saw hairy legs in the next bathroom stall and even though there was a scheduled time for male or female shower use, I dressed behind the shower curtain. After a couple of weeks of overwhelming orientations and mind-boggling reading assignments, I was too tired to care.

Biochemistry, statistics, medical/surgical labs, and clinical rotations threatened me each morning, and denied me sleep at the end of the day. I drove home on weekends to be with Sydney and Pascha and to catch up on housekeeping and laundry while I listened to lectures on headphones. I rewrote my own notes and read them into a tape recorder and I slept with the words seeping into my dreams, hoping I would pass yet another exam.

There was little time for fun or holidays, but as Halloween approached, the students arranged a dance in the dorm lobby. My roommate helped me climb into a box and we stuffed a teddy bear head through the top and draped a long bathrobe over the box. With some IV tubing snaking through the robe into the box I was able to enjoy the refreshments but I didn't speak. I danced with several guys. One of my young partners, an oriental student, kept asking me what my name was. I danced with him, and flirted with the teddy bear head but never spoke. A couple of weeks later when Sydney and Pascha were visiting me on campus we went to the gym to exercise. My dance partner was handing out towels and I couldn't resist telling him that I was the lady in the box. Sydney, Pascha and I thought it was a great joke, but the embarrassed student bowed repeatedly, apologizing to his elders.

I survived the first year, and Pascha and I returned to Camp Taloali for the summer. Francis was swollen from the prednisone he needed. His ankles hung over his shoes, and he had what could have been mistaken for a beer belly. The Blue Cross insurance policy denied coverage for his pre-existing condition. He would have to apply again after a waiting period. Meanwhile, he had no way to pay for his health care. I made an appointment with the gastroenterology professor at the university. I told him about my son's illness and his financial situation. I offered to do housecleaning, child care or work in his office if he would see Francis. He took Francis on as a patient and during the next three years we never received a bill from that kind doctor. He never collected on my offer to do free housework or babysitting. Dr. Emmet Keefe wound his way through the long lines of medical, dental and nursing students to give me a hug when I graduated.

Gardner, who had been in Denver, was back in Oregon. He came to the university to visit me with a constrictor snake in a briefcase. He claimed he had a part time job in a pet store and that he was taming the snake to make it more marketable. The snake was not welcome in the dorm, so Gardner and I went to a restaurant .to eat. I couldn't help but giggle about the secret contents of the briefcase when the waitress came to take our order. It seemed like old times to be with Gardner and wondering where his snakes were. He was thirty-one and in some kind of trouble again. He said he was worried he would be sentenced as a habitual criminal, and he didn't think anyone would believe his side of the story. That was the last time any of us heard from him for over twenty years.

And then, more pounding at my front door. Francis again.

"Mom, I almost killed myself." He was scared, lonely, and depressed. He had decided to let his truck go back to the bank for what he owed on it. He had to quit working and didn't know how he would get by or if he should even try. I lived in fear that he would kill himself, but I also feared that I all my emotions would be drained before that happened. He threw away the picture of himself accepting the presidency of the Explorer Scout Deputy Sheriff Program in Great Falls. I dug it out the garbage and put it away.

The yoyo continued. Francis had great news. A different doctor said he was stable and doing so well a liver transplant could be put on the back burner. I won a lottery drawn among 38 nursing students. I was one of five seniors assigned to the NICU for clinical rotation in pediatrics. I hoped I might even get to make a run with the helicopter crew.

Sydney and Pascha moved to Portland and we crammed into campus housing for my senior year. I liked going home after classes to a somewhat normal family life.

My psychiatric nursing rotation was at the Dougy Center and was one of those serendipity events people talk about. The Dougy Center was the first official children's bereavement center in the United States; Dr. Elizabeth Kubler-Ross cut the ribbons at the grand opening. I had attended a lecture by Dr. Kubler-Ross the year before, and when I left the auditorium I knew what I wanted to be when I grew up. At The Dougy Center I had an opportunity to work with children who had lost a loved one from illness or accident, or from suicide or homicide. I took graduate entrance exams, and applied to graduate nursing programs with a goal to become a mental health practitioner, working in the field of childhood bereavement.

I graduated with honors, and received the Dorothy Johnson Award for patient advocacy. Sydney bought me a bright blue Suzuki with a canvas top, and for two days after graduation I made sure everyone on campus knew it was mine. We put balloons on the antenna and I honked up and down University Hill where most of the students knew the old lady from Montana.

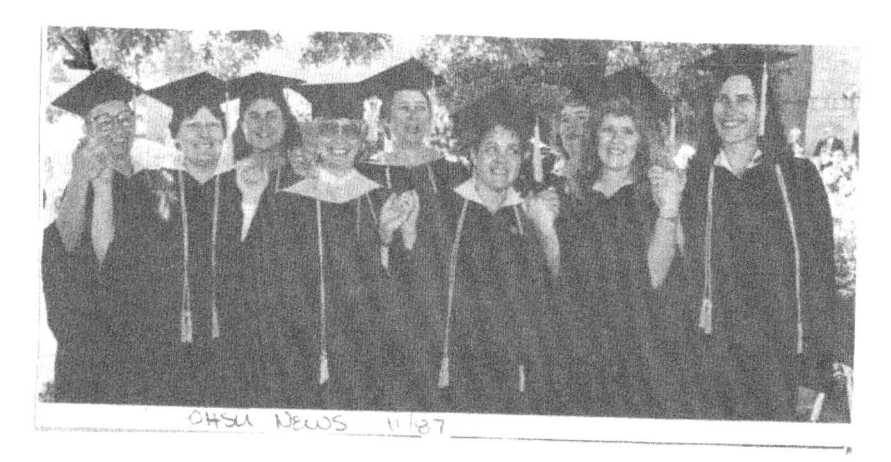

Graduate school and a TA position at Montana State University in Bozeman were waiting for me. Francis, Pascha, Sydney and I settled into the small university town and we snooped through farmer's market on weekends, explored canyons and streams and I contacted my brothers Paul and Walt who lived in nearby towns. Walt and his wife came to Bozeman for a reunion visit, but Paul wasn't ready to meet the little sister they had left behind forty years earlier. Margaret sent her congratulations, and said our mother would have been very proud. Margaret told me Mother wanted her to be a nurse. I was the first person in my family, and Sydney's, to earn a college degree.

Graduate school was challenging but rewarding until the day I took a call from the medical school in Baylor, Texas. Francis had an appointment to go there to have an evaluation for a liver transplant. Blue Cross medical insurance would insure him for most of the $250,000 he needed for a transplant and Francis had his airline tickets.

The string of my yoyo existence broke on the fourth of December when a person in the accounting office at Baylor called to remind me that Francis would need to pay the deductible when he arrived. He needed $70,000 before he could be admitted. I just hung up the phone. I sat down and wept, and any anger that was left from my awakening rage melted into despair. I couldn't find a way to tell Francis. We had never seen $70,000 in our lives. Francis took the news quietly and retired to his room. I took prescription drugs to maintain in school until Christmas break. We poured over material at the library researching possible grants; then slept and cried some more. Francis threatened to die just to show people how unjust things were. His conversations flipped from finding an apartment in Great Falls, to suicide. His best buddy from Oregon stopped by on his way to a military assignment in Greece. Tim was in the Navy and living the dream the two of them had hoped to share. When he left it was snowing softly and Francis hung onto the car door, talking and saying goodbye, but not letting his friend go. Then he came into the living room; walked to his room and shut the door. When relatives heard we needed money, the cards and letters stopped.

When Francis developed a dental problem and needed a root canal I told him he should just have the tooth pulled, and then I realized what I was really saying. The evening news showed a mass murder of a family somewhere and our family counted six livers gone to waste. We wondered if we could buy burial insurance and if not we wondered if any of our extended family would help us bury our son.

I dropped out of school, and we moved to Great Falls to be near a larger hospital. The move was devastating to Pascha. He had a wonderful teacher in Bozeman and had made friends his age. He walked across the front yard of our house in Great Falls each morning on his way to school with his head down. Each step was slow and looked heavy, as though he had the weight of the world on his small shoulders.

Francis found an efficiency apartment, and because he was feeling pretty good, we all went into a shared denial. Kathleen became my rock. She was there to listen, but didn't try to cheer me up. She had already buried a son and knew the futility of empty words of comfort. My sister showed her age with slumped shoulders and gnarled fingers

In the fall of 1986, when Francis was 25, Medicaid made a determination that they would only pay for liver transplants for individuals under 18 years old. Francis's mood darkened; now he owned the rage. He resented my future, and he hated Pascha's youth. We learned that humans were not blessed when God gave them knowledge of their own mortality and I learned anticipatory death is a misnomer.

CHAPTER 18—CAMP FRANCIS

Yellowstone Park was on fire and it seemed most of Montana was burning that summer of 1988. When I stopped at Francis's apartment to pick up his laundry I pulled up his window shades and the big sky was obscured by brown smoke. I could taste the acrid air and it seemed like the end of the world had come. Then, a rare August snowstorm put out the fires and autumn in Montana was as it should be; clear, crisp and colorful. Winter didn't return to Great Falls until the end of January.

Then, gray, heavy clouds hung close to the 8th floor of the hospital where Francis was hospitalized with undiagnosed headaches. He picked at invisible things in the air around his bed. After his first stroke, one of his eyes wandered about on a search and destroy mission. I leaned over, looked right into his eyes and asked him what he was thinking about. He struggled to speak.

"How beautiful you are."

The words were slurred and that was the last time he spoke, except for obscenities. Before the stroke, the doctors said, "severe migraines." Now, nurses whispered to me, "Get him out of Great Falls." How? I wondered.

I screamed when I accused the doctor of treating my son as though he was terminal, and the doctor screamed back that Francis was terminal. I called the hospital chaplain, and asked if he could help me. He had the answer and the power, maybe the higher power, because he found a fixed-wing jet that could take Francis and me to Portland. But first I had to find a doctor that would accept Francis as a patient. I called our dear Dr. Keefe.

I climbed into the plane behind the stretcher and a nurse who would go with us. Pascha and Sydney waved goodbye to us as the plane taxied for take off; the plane climbed through the clouds hanging over Great Falls and my fear that we might be too late lifted a bit as the sky cleared. When Mount Hood came into our view, Francis and I shared tears of relief. I walked behind the stretcher as it rolled through the halls of my alma mater, Oregon Health Science University and I felt powerful. I pulled my fist down in a victory sign and said to myself, "Yes!" I had saved my son. I had accomplished the impossible. With no money, no insurance, no family help, I had commandeered an airplane!

The doctors in Portland did a spinal tap the next day and found that Francis had contracted a rare fungal disease. He had cryptococcal meningitis and he may have got it from a parakeet we had at home because the medications he took to fight his disease lowered his immune system.

Francis endured severe side effects from the medication used to kill the fungus, but some days were too much for him. Then he bit through the IV tubing, letting the medicine run onto the floor. He cursed the restraints that kept his hands tied to the bedrails after that.

Family trickled in and out of his room for over a month. Our hopes for his survival rose and fell with his response to therapies. Daniel, the oldest brother that Francis had never met, came from Seattle and Patty came from Spokane to be with us. Stephen lived in Portland and was at his brother's bedside as much as possible.   Danette drove up from Salem several times. She pulled the window shades up when I pulled them down and when I gave Francis a bath, she gave him a better one. She parted his hair on the "other "side and in many other ways she said, without words, "It's your fault. You were a bad mother."

I owned my guilt. It was mine, but so was Francis, and I told her I had given him life and I had the right to see him through to his death.

He looked like a bronze statue as his colored changed. His cheeks sunk deep into his face, and his eyelids darkened, but he looked peaceful for the first time in a long while. The fluids in his urine bag turned deep red, bloody; his thighs turned purple as blood seeped from his veins and then I knew it was time; no more insulin. As he slipped into a coma I held his hand. Sydney and I took his turns at the bedside throughout the night. Francis made slow movements with his hand acknowledging our presence. With his favorite music playing, and his siblings gathered around, I took him in my arms and rocked him, as I shushed him away.

Family and friends took care of the services. Sydney, Pascha and I took the train back to Montana. Patty and Danny returned to their lives in Washington and Stephen stayed on in Portland. Danette did come to the funeral, but she quietly slipped away before I realized she was gone. Once again she had slipped out of my life, this time taking my granddaughter with her.

Stephen came in the spring and we put the ashes in the cemetery where Francis's baby sister was buried. At the graveside Stephen said; "My brother was such a jerk, and we fought all the time. God I'm going to miss him."

I went back to work at the psychiatric unit of the Deaconess Hospital which was on the south end of the building and everyday I looked out the windows, past the prairie, to the cemetery where my children were and wondered why I wasn't with them. Pascha was eleven; the same age I had been when I was forced to face my future as a motherless child. I had to keep breathing.

Grief is hard work. Sydney cursed the circumstances, and wished he had done things differently. I was afraid to grieve. I didn't want Francis to become a distant memory like Topsy had. I could still feel his presence all around me.

I tried to go back to Portland to continue my graduate work and foolishly accepted a nursing job on the unit where Francis had died. Meanwhile, Stephen had entered therapy to deal with the sexual abuse he and his brother had endured and we spent some quality time supporting each other in our pain. I returned to Montana for Pascha's birthday and I thanked God for my extra son who filled some of the holes in my heart. He seemed to be ok with a part-time mother and he was busy with football, tuba practice, the swim team and a computer class.

My professor in psych nursing asked me to submit a grant to the National Institute of Mental Health. The deadline was that afternoon. I wrote a brief summary of my plans to return to Montana to work as children's grief therapist on a piece of scrap paper. The grant would not only pay my tuition and books, but would pay my living expenses. It was an outstanding piece of luck that I got the grant. While I was home for Thanksgiving, our neighbor, Pascha's babysitter died; right after the funeral I learned my brother Walt had lung cancer that had spread to his brain. It seemed that Dr. Taylor's observation that I was waiting around for the next funeral was prophetic. As Christmas drew near, I couldn't find any joy in the season and I resented the happiness around me. Grief came in waves, and my stomach lurched up like I was on a rollercoaster.

I returned to school in January and Oregon rained. The rat-a-tat-tat, on the window kept rhythm with my heartbeat. I feared my heart would stop, and then I feared it wouldn't. I walked out of class in February and packed my things and climbed on the train pointed toward Montana.

I washed walls and curtains and made bread, and I stopped crying. My friends in Great Falls were glad to see me, and my enemies were happy that I had failed. I tried to go back to school the next fall. I packed my books in my jeep, and crossed the mountains. My anxiety increased with each mile and a little west of Spokane I spun the car around, and like a horse with the bit in his teeth bound for the barn, I didn't stop until I was home. Pascha was walking down the sidewalk after school when he saw me sitting on the porch; he ran the rest of the way. He asked why I came back and I said, "I thought maybe you needed a mother this year."

He sat down beside me and slipped his arm around my waist.

Seasons come and go, and families have their seasons too. Patty's girls in Spokane were getting married and starting families. Sydney, with Shirley—who was by then a widow—on one arm, and me on the other, became the patriarch of our mixed families and escorted the two grandmothers at their weddings. Stephen came back to Great Falls and married a Montana girl and Danette and Angela came for that wedding. Gardner, lost to all of us, was unaware that his brother had died and that he was an uncle.

Allen Wolfelt, a well-known bereavement therapist in Colorado says that mourning is grief gone public. As I progressed through my own mourning, I found a way to lead others out of the lonely place called grief.

The nurses were discussing a large endowment that was given to the pediatric unit at the hospital in Great Falls. They were complaining about the way the money was being used. I said, "Well, I know what I would do with some of it."

That flippant statement was the birth of a program called MYMOM'S.

As a class project I had written a children's book about death and dying. The narrator was a little boy who told his friends that his mom knew all about death and dying and she would tell them about it. Throughout the story the little boy says, "Let's go to MYMOM'S and ask her." Hence the name for a program that would help children and adolescents talk about death and dying.

With a handful of friends and volunteers I began offering bi-monthly support programs for children who were grieving. I wrote proposals and made a pest of myself at hospital meetings in pursuit of both financial and professional support for the program I was developing.

One of the volunteers, who worked with at risk adolescents, had reserved a spot at a summer camp and he wasn't going to use it. He suggested we hold a camp for grieving children. I thought about my experience at Camp Taloali in Oregon with the deaf community and thought I had the skills to manage a camp.

The first Camp Francis was held in June of 1993. The camp experience, four days in the wilderness, was offered free to children and their families who had experienced the death of someone close to them. The volunteers and I combed the community in search of donations. Camper shirts had the wrong year on them and didn't match. Teddy bears from volunteer bedrooms and the Goodwill became camper buddies. A retired couple scraped up some family-style meals from donated groceries and another retired volunteer provided chopped firewood for the lodge. Heavy rains caused the nearby creek to rise enough that evacuation was almost certain, but our soggy group made it to the closing ceremonies and released message balloons into a clear Montana sky while music on an amplifier rang out across the pastures.

The director of the hospital's hospice program took a personal interest in the MYMOM'S program and through her efforts I was able to sell the program and the camp to the hospital. I was hired to oversee the project. I brought in an expert from the Dougy Center to train a handpicked group of volunteers. Nurses, psychologists, social workers, chaplains, teachers, and others interested individuals spent four days learning about how children grieve and how we could help the children.

I visited the Dougy Center to learn how to develop the program and I attended seminars and workshops around the United States to learn the latest theories in children's grief therapy. The MYMOM'S program began offering grief specific groups. We had a group for children who had lost a loved one to suicide or homicide, or had lost a sibling, or a parent, or grandparent. During those gatherings the children sat in a welcoming circle and passed around a "talking stick." "My name is Susie, or John, and I came to MYMOM'S because my—sister, mother, friend, etc.—died. The group leaders provided media for the children to express their grief. The kids painted pictures of their loved one or of their feelings, they made up and sang songs, they danced for the group to show how grief felt, they threw ice cubes at a brick wall and stomped on bubble packaging to kill cancer cells and sometimes they sat in a corner with a stuffed animal and cried. We put stars that glowed in the dark on the ceiling of our room and each child had a star with the loved ones name on it. At the end of the meeting we dimmed the lights and held hands while we sang a closing song and looked at the stars that shone done on us. One very little boy who had watched his mother kill herself talked about the horrific incident too much. The teacher at his school called us for help because he kept telling his story to his young peers. One of the volunteers, a child psychologist brought an old typewriter and he and the boy wrote the story and made a book and the little boy stopped talking about it at school. We took the grief support program to the high schools and students who had experienced a recent loss were excused from class once a week to attend

A team of volunteers formed what we called Wednesday's Child. Those volunteers wore beepers and would respond to a request from the hospital, the ambulance, or to a home where a child was with someone dying. We also offered escort service for children at funerals if it was requested by the family.

I wrote a manual for other communities to refer to as they developed similar camps and those manuals were sold at conferences in Seattle, Boston, and Cleveland and through bereavement magazines. Each year graduating campers became our "word of mouth" advertisement and camp attendance grew. Many of the teens who came to camp came back as mentors and teen counselors. Youngsters came to Camp Francis scared and reluctant to acknowledge their loss and their feelings about loss. When it came time to say their goodbyes at the end of the session the same campers begged their parents to let them come back the next summer.

Native American volunteers showed the campers how to make Dream Catchers and volunteer clowns drew happy faces over tears. As the community learned about camp, volunteers brought horses for the kids to ride or baked cakes for a birthday cake walk. A family with many adopted children donated their time and talent to bring their sound system and musical talent to camp and a professional band called Pollo Loco brought the makings of a dance in the lodge for the "day off" that was held in the middle of the week. We once held an old fashioned box social and a real auctioneer volunteered her talents to auction off the lunches made in our kitchen. New camp shirts, hats and shorts with the hospital logo and colors were added to the tradition after the hospital bought the program and a camp flag, white, with the words "Camp Francis" in turquoise, waves above the lodge each summer.

Camp Francis was featured on television and in local news stories. Reporters came to camp for the final ceremony each year. We had a traditional homemade parade in which the children marched with banners and instruments to declare their plans to march back into life and love. Each year a celebrity came to give the children their graduation certificates. Those celebrities included Deputy Sheriffs who came with their sirens and lights flashing, Search and Rescue dogs who demonstrated how they find lost people, and local news people. One year a well known bereavement author, Darcy Simms was able to join us because Horizon Airlines donated tickets.

In 1999 the surprise celebrity for the closing ceremonies at Camp Francis was Marc Racicot, the governor of Montana. A helicopter circled the campgrounds while curious campers craned their necks to watch, and then with a chop, chop, chop it landed softly onto the baseball field, and the Governor stepped out. He presented each camper with their certificate, and then he sat down in a circle with the children and shared tears with them. I felt so proud of my success in bringing the governor to camp that I wrote a letter to Colin Powell, the then leader of America's Promise and asked him to come the next year. He wasn't able to be at camp but he wrote a nice letter of commendation.

Camp Francis, an old camp ground in central Montana, is really a place in the hearts of children who learned to express their pain and dared to march back into life. For fifteen years, the flag has flown over the campgrounds. Francis' spirit is personified in the noise of children learning to express their grief.

CONCLUSION

I am the matriarch now, the old one, as the natives in Montanans say. I carry the genetic defects, and I rue my past mistakes. My life has been as broad as the Big Sky country that I have called home. Now I welcome the Chinooks that have melted my many winters of discontent. I look toward the mountains, those granite sentinels that stand between forest and prairie, still promising wanderers a better life, just over the pass, and I know I do not need to make that trek again.

In my twilight years I watch the sun slip reluctantly behind the Rockies and I know that the dust will settle and the orange glow of the skyline will fade into the color of a cowboy's jeans. Then, the rhinestone heavens and the Northern lights will set the silent stage for tomorrow's dreams.

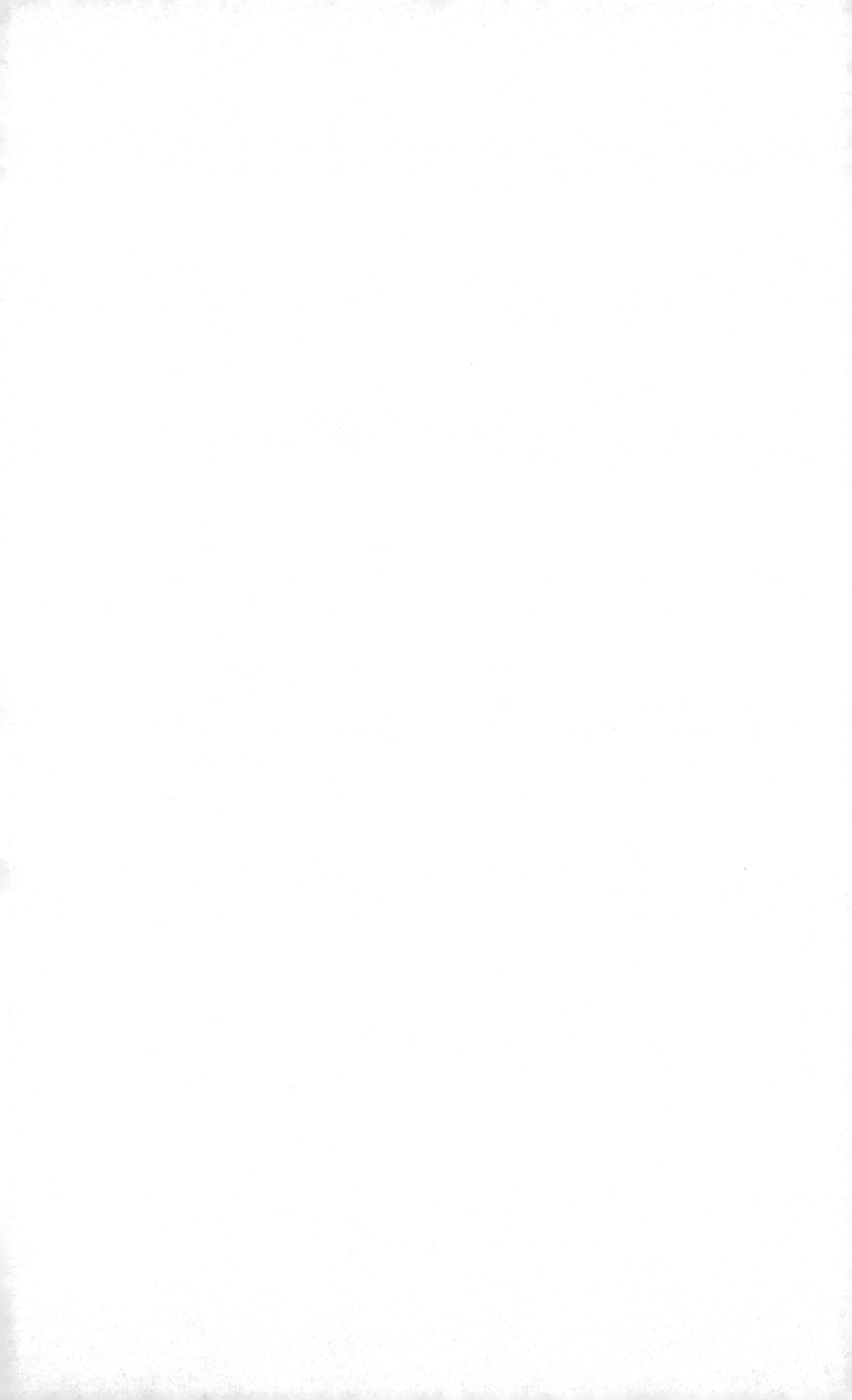

EPILOGUE

Many of the people in my story are gone now. My brothers and sister have died and although there are nieces and nephews still living in Montana I am not in contact with them. My sister joined our family for holidays and we developed an adult relationship before she died. The death of her estranged son probably contributed to her failing health. Her daughter Diane who lives in Utah has been the niece that all old aunties should be lucky enough to have. She remembers everyone in our family with handwritten birthday notes and keeps me up to date about her two sons and their families.

I don't think there are many Johnson relatives left and if there are, I do not know where they live. Aunt Eula spent her last years at a nursing home in Fort Benton and captured the hearts of all who worked there.

Life twisted around in its funny way and Lynn Fontaine's grandchildren came through the bereavement program when their dad Michael died. I had been with their grandmother the day the doctor told her Michael would not live past his second year. I was not in Montana when Lynn died but I heard he had a huge funeral at the church he attended regularly.

Daniel Banich did get to spend some time with Patty and Gardner after they grew into adulthood but Danette refused his request to attend her wedding and Francis and Stephen had no memories of him. He spent his last years, as a hermit digging for gold in the Arizona desert. The cause of his death was never determined. His son Daniel, who went by Mitchell after his adoption refused to acknowledge his birth name of Banich. He lived with his biological mother, Shirley, until he died from an embolism in 2006.

George Holly married twice after our divorce and I heard he died of liver cancer in 1977.

Nick and Mary Holoboff celebrated their fiftieth wedding anniversary and lived over ten more years together before Mary died and Nick went into an assisted living facility. He died in 2003. Sydney's siblings, with the exception of his widowed sister, Molly, will probably celebrate their golden anniversaries in the next few years.

Although Sydney and I may not live long enough to celebrate a fiftieth anniversary, we have been married for thirty-two years and Patty and Greg are close behind. They have been together thirty-one year and just welcomed their first great-grandchild.

Danette and Steve live in Oregon and have four grandchildren. Stephen and Cindy have made their home in the northwest corner of Montana and have two children still in school. Pascha and my youngest grandchild are in Missoula.

I saved the update on Gardner for the last because it is so special. For over twenty years none of us heard from him and we began to think he may have drifted out of the country and died somehow because even when he was in prison in his younger years he always called me for Christmas or Mother's Day. Then one day in 2005 the phone rang and there he was. He said he never called because he wasn't anyone I would have wanted to know during the years he was missing.

I have come to know him now and his rebirth is a wonderful gift in my old age. The next year Gardner received a similar gift when his son, Shane called him after locating his lost dad on the internet. Shane brought his wife and Gardner's two grandchildren to our Thanksgiving table in 2006.

My dear friend Kathy and I are celebrating fifty years of friendship and sharing our blended families' milestones. I am a Catholic now, and today, after church, I am going to stop by Kathy's. After all these years, her coffee pot is still on.

About the Author

Carol Holoboff, a native Montanan, grew up in the Golden Triangle area of central Montana. She attended schools in Great Falls, Helena, and Sunburst. She received a Bachelor's Degree in Nursing from the Oregon Health Science University and attended graduate schools in both Montana and Oregon. She is the founder of Camp Francis, the first residential camp for bereaved children and considers that her legacy to her home town of Great Falls. Carol also worked closely with state and federal officials at the site of an environmental disaster in Libby, Montana and as a reporter for a local newspaper. She writes a column called "The Calico Pen." She currently lives in Great Falls and enjoys traveling with her husband Sydney and their two dogs, Sadie Mae and W. T. Beuford.

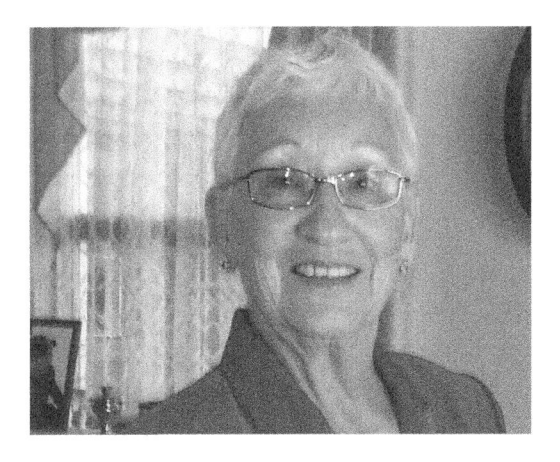

KEYNOTE A white-trash to white-collar saga of a wild Montana child who overcomes her destiny and in a pied piper fashion shows others a better way.

ENDORESMENTS
An unforgettable look at a family fractured by mental and physical illness and sexual violence. Carol Holoboff unsparingly details her journey from neglected childhood (including stints in an orphanage and a Montana reform school, through failed marriages and a volunteer stay in the Oregon mental institution made famous by One Flew Over the Cuckoo's Nest, to her role as family matriarch. A riveting read. Ruth McLaughlin, M.F.A.

"Growing up in the west, under big open skies, picking out candy in small neighborhood grocery stores and weekend rodeos, is in itself a great adventure. Carol Holoboff's book artfully captures the essence of the west as it threads along the dirt roads of her native Montana and winds through a life marked by both commonality and great surprise. The Bastard Tree is one of those rare books you will glue yourself to, one you'll read in a few long, pleasurable settings. "
Gordon Sullivan, author of Saving Homewaters.

"Truly the author has turned trials and tribulations into triumph. Her life experiences have given her a deep empathy for the trouble of others, and her work with bereaved children is commendable. "Chris Cauble, Riverbend Publishing

Made in the USA
Coppell, TX
04 April 2024

30902590R00121